Gastroesophageal Reflux Disease - A Growing Concern

Edited by Jianyuan Chai

Published in London, United Kingdom

Gastroesophageal Reflux Disease - A Growing Concern
http://dx.doi.org/10.5772/intechopen.100999
Edited by Jianyuan Chai

Contributors
Ladan Panahi, Anthony Wilks, George Udeani, Salim Surani, Ljiljana Širić, Marinela Rosso, Aleksandar Včev, I Dewa Nyoman Wibawa, Ni Wayan Wina Dharmesti, Jianyuan Chai, Xianmei Meng, Zaim Gashi, Arjeta Gashi, Fadil Sherifi

First published in London, United Kingdom, 2023 by IntechOpen
IntechOpen is the global imprint of INTECHOPEN LIMITED, registered in England and Wales, registration number: 11086078, 5 Princes Gate Court, London, SW7 2QJ, United Kingdom

British Library Cataloguing-in-Publication Data
A catalogue record for this book is available from the British Library

Additional hard and PDF copies can be obtained from orders@intechopen.com

Gastroesophageal Reflux Disease - A Growing Concern
Edited by Jianyuan Chai
p. cm.
Print ISBN 978-1-80355-957-5
Online ISBN 978-1-80355-958-2
eBook (PDF) ISBN 978-1-80355-959-9

Meet the editor

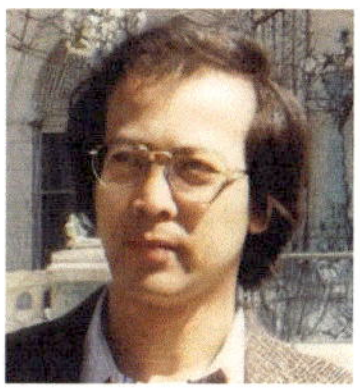

Dr. Chai received his Ph.D. in Biology from the City University of New York in 1998 and completed his postdoctoral training in molecular medicine at Harvard University in 2001. Then he served the Department of Veterans Affairs of the United States as a Principal Investigator (2002-2016), in affiliation with the School of Medicine, University of California, Irvine, USA. Currently, he is a professor at Baotou Medical College, China. Dr. Chai has published dozens of research articles on various subjects including zoology, cardiovascular biology, gastroenterology, and cancer biology. His current research interest is esophageal cancer.

Contents

Preface

Gastroesophageal reflux disease (GERD) is the most common digestive disorder worldwide. Despite efforts made over the years in GERD treatment and prevention, GERD incidence is still growing steadily. According to the latest report, GERD increased by 77.53% globally during 1990–2019, from 440 million to 780 million. Most of the cases came from India and China, the two most populated countries, accounting for 180 million and 80 million cases, respectively. Due to the lack of a unifying standard for diagnosis, the actual number of GERD sufferers is likely much higher. Based on a recent meta-analysis, GERD potentially affects 0.9–1.1 billion people worldwide, which is about 14% of the current global population. The impact of GERD on word health and economy is great. In Europe, for example, GERD caused a 26% reduction in productivity, costing employers approximately 4.4 billion dollars in 2018.

GERD mainly affects two organs: the esophagus and the stomach. Although these two organs are neighboring parts of the digestive tract and both are involved in transporting food from the mouth to the intestine for digestion and absorption, they constitute a one-way street. Food can only go from the esophagus to the stomach, otherwise, it will cause damage to the epithelial lining of the esophagus because the ingested food becomes highly acidic once reaching the stomach. The squamous epithelium in the esophagus is not made to stand such a highly acidic condition and, as a result, esophagitis develops. When these reflux episodes take place again and again, the esophageal lining gradually changes from squamous to columnar, becoming the intestinal-like phenotype, which is called Barrett's Esophagus. When this happens, the patient is 400 times more likely to develop esophageal cancer.

The lower esophageal sphincter (LES) is a muscular structure sitting between the esophagus and the stomach that prevents the stomach content from going into the esophagus. Therefore, anything that interrupts LES function is a potential cause of GERD. Obesity or overweight is the number one factor. The excessive weight in the abdominal region puts constant pressure on the stomach, forcing the stomach content to break the LES barrier and erupt into the esophagus, causing esophagitis. Other factors include eating habits, lifestyle, taking certain drugs, esophageal or gastric motility weakness, and so on. Some common food and drinks (e.g., coffee, tea, soda, juices, alcoholic beverages, chocolates, tomatoes, high-fat or high-calorie food, or spicy food) can create occasional GERD episodes in healthy individuals or worsen the condition of GERD patients. Many medications can also interfere with the LES function and result in GERD symptoms, such as nitrates, calcium channel blockers, anticholinergic drugs, benzodiazepines, nitroglycerin, albuterol, antidepressants, glucagon, and non-steroidal anti-inflammatory drugs (NSAIDs).

For these reasons, the current strategies for GERD management and prevention mainly rely on changing eating habits, modifying lifestyle, suppressing gastric acid secretion, and surgically restoring LES function. However, none of these have achieved satisfaction so far. GERD incidence is still growing day by day, year after year. Why? Let's look at these strategies one by one.

First, let's ask ourselves a question: can we really quit eating and drinking coffee, tea, soda, juice, alcohol, chocolate, tomatoes, and high-fat, high-calorie, or spicy food? Will we still be able to enjoy our lives if we eliminate these foods and beverages from our daily diet? We have been eating and drinking this stuff for generation after generation, for as long as we can remember. Giving all these up is impossible for most of us and thus we must think of a new way to deal with the problem of GERD.

Now, let's look at acid-suppressive drugs. From antacids to H2 blockers (famotidine and cimetidine) to proton pump inhibitors (omeprazole, lansoprazole, esomeprazole, pantoprazole, dexlansoprazole, and rabeprazole), the basic idea is to lower or neutralize gastric acid secretion and thereby reduce the esophageal damage caused by refluxes. First, we must know that pathological GERD is not due to acid secretion. We need gastric acid to sterilize our ingested food and create a suitable environment for enzymatic digestion. Acid suppression will definitely interfere with these purposes. Growing evidence has shown multiple side effects in association with taking acid-suppressing drugs, including decreased absorption of vitamins/minerals, susceptibility to infections, bone fracture, and even greater risk of developing cancer. Once they stop taking these drugs, 70%–100% of patients will experience GERD episodes again. We must think of a new way to deal with the GERD problem.

Laparoscopic Nissen Fundoplication is now considered to be the gold standard for the surgical treatment of GERD. This is a great idea because this procedure intends to solve the problem by restoring LES function so that gastric contents will be unable to get into the esophagus. However, this technique has not gained success as expected. After surgery, many patients have developed postoperative adverse symptoms such as bloating, dysphagia, and belching. As a result, 62% of patients had to go back to taking acid-suppressive drugs. We must think of a new way to deal with the GERD problem.

Compared to all these therapeutic ideas, modifying lifestyle seems the most achievable. We can do more exercises to control our weight, we can avoid lying down right after meals, we can raise our pillows before sleep, and so on. These actions are typically easy to implement; however, will they eliminate GERD? Unfortunately, the answer is no. We must think of a new way to deal with the GERD problem.

This book provides a comprehensive overview of GERD and discusses the various techniques employed to relieve associated symptoms.

Jianyuan Chai
Professor,
Inner Mongolia Institute of Digestive Diseases,
Baotou Medical College,
Baotou, China

Chapter 1

Introductory Chapter: Do We Really Know GERD?

Xianmei Meng and Jianyuan Chai

1. Introduction

Gastroesophageal reflux disease (GERD), commonly known as heartburn, has been one of the most prevalent digestive disorders for the past few decades. Despite various definitions in different parts of the world, GERD generally refers to the effortless movement of stomach contents into the esophagus causing troublesome symptoms, typically a burning sensation in the chest, which may radiate toward the neck, throat, and the back, inducing pain. Chronic GERD can lead to several complications, including erosive esophagitis, esophageal strictures, and esophageal epithelial transformation into Barrett's Esophagus (squamous epithelium turning into columnar epithelium), a precancerous condition to adenocarcinoma. Therefore, early diagnosis and proper treatment are critical for the prevention of these potential complications and malignancy. Due to its popularity, GERD has not only deteriorated the quality of life for many people all over the world, but it has also brought up tremendous economic pressure on many countries and regions. European Digestive Health Summit 2018 reported a 26% reduction in productivity across Europe because of GERD, costing employers ~$4.4 billion [1]. In the United States, the expenses on GERD were estimated to be at least $24 billion/year [2].

2. How many people are affected by GERD? we do not know

There has never been a unifying definition for GERD; consequently, GERD diagnosis has never had a gold standard. Mostly, it is made based on questionnaires in combination with a few additional examinations and tests, including responsiveness to acid-suppressive drugs, esophagogastroduodenoscopy (EGD), and ambulatory reflux monitoring. Weekly heartburn or acid regurgitation is the first indicator of GERD. Heartburn refers to a retrosternal burning sensation that typically occurs after a meal or when in a reclined position, and regurgitation is the backflow of stomach contents into the mouth or throat. However, some GERD patients are asymptomatic. As reported in Europe, 44–46% of the patients with Barrett's Esophagus never showed any sign of heartburn or acid regurgitation [3]. Among those presenting these symptoms, on the other hand, a significant proportion is caused by other pathological conditions rather than GERD. As evidenced in the United Kingdom, only 66% of the patients with heartburn or regurgitation were confirmed to be GERD by endoscopic examination and 24-hr pH monitoring [4]. Likewise, among the real GERD patients, only 49% ever experienced heartburn or acid regurgitation. Therefore, having GERD symptoms does not necessarily mean having GERD.

In addition to heartburn and acid regurgitation, other less common discomforts can also be connected to GERD, including burping, hiccups, water brash, dysphagia, odynophagia, chronic cough, chronic laryngitis, asthma, nausea, and vomiting. However, these symptoms are often seen in other disorders as well, such as eosinophilic esophagitis [5], functional dyspepsia [6], gastroparesis [7], and coronary artery disease [8].

Nowadays, many acid-suppressive drugs are accessible without prescription. Taking these medications, especially Proton Pump Inhibitors (PPI), can conceal GERD-induced esophageal abnormalities. In such cases, even EGD cannot always identify GERD, but ambulatory esophageal pH monitoring can help to correlate the symptoms with pathological acid exposure. Barium radiographs can also be helpful in the detection of esophagitis, esophageal strictures, hiatal hernia, and esophageal tumors.

All of these factors often make GERD diagnosis difficult. As a result, the exact number of people affected by GERD remains to be a mystery. We can only guess how many GERD people are out there, based on the published data. A recent meta-analysis using the data from January 1, 1947, to June 30, 2018, might be able to give us a general idea. According to this study, the global GERD population is likely to be around 1.03 billion (920,661,200–1,148,796,172), representing 13.98% of the current human population on this planet. To make matters worse, the number is still growing year after year.

3. What causes GERD? we do not know

Since the backflow of gastric contents into the esophagus is harmful, to prevent this to happen, the esophagus is anatomically separated from the stomach by the gastroesophageal barrier that consists of two tough muscular components, the lower esophageal sphincter (LES) and the diaphragm. The LES is the 3–4 cm (in adults) distal portion of the esophagus penetrating the diaphragm through the hiatus and entering the abdominal cavity where it connects to the stomach. The diaphragm keeps the esophagus and the stomach in the thoracic cavity and the abdominal cavity separately. The LES and the diaphragm are anchored to each other by the phrenoesophageal ligament so that these two components contract coordinately to prevent the backflow of the stomach contents into the esophagus. For this reason, anything disturbing the function of the gastroesophageal barrier is a potential cause of GERD.

Over the years, many factors have been evaluated for a possible connection with the disease but no one is singled out. Based on the statistical significance, the top five reasons for GERD occurrence are listed as follows.

1. **Overweight/obesity**. Body weight has been commonly recognized as a major contributor to GERD development. The excessive body fat, especially around the abdominal region, puts constant pressure on the stomach, squeezing the gastric fluid to break the gastroesophageal barrier entering the esophageal lumen frequently, damaging the esophageal lining. According to a meta-analysis [9], GERD was detected in 6.64% of the people with a body mass index (BMI) below 18.5, but in 22.63% of the individuals with a BMI above 30, which is the baseline defined for obesity.

2. **Hiatal hernia**. The hiatus is the small opening in the center of the diaphragm, which allows the esophagus to pass through from the thoracic cavity into the abdominal cavity where it connects to the stomach. In the condition of hiatal hernia, an upper portion of the stomach along with the LES bulges through the hiatus into the thoracic cavity, making the stomach contents easily get into the esophagus. A German study found hiatal hernia in 95% of GERD patients [10].

3. **Frequent transient LES relaxation**. Normally, the LES is conically contracted at rest to produce a concentric occlusion, keeping the stomach contents from backing up. When we are swallowing, the LES relaxes for a few seconds to allow the ingested object to enter the stomach. However, several activities can potentially increase the frequency and duration (> 20 seconds) of the transient LES relaxation, for example, smoking, drinking, and taking certain medications. Many medications are known to cause more frequent or extended transient LES relaxation, such as nitrates, calcium channel blockers, anticholinergic drugs, benzodiazepines, nitroglycerin, albuterol, antidepressants, glucagon, and non-steroidal anti-inflammatory drugs (NSAIDs) [11, 12]. Based on a meta-analysis [9], 24.47% of the NSAID users were found to have GERD, compared with 17.34% of the non-users. Interestingly, however, the study also showed that drinking coffee, tea, or carbonated beverages all increase the odds of GERD, but drinking alcoholic beverages does not seem to be a significant factor [9]. Overall, frequent transient LES relaxation is connected to 48–73% of GERD symptoms [13].

4. **Impairment of esophageal motility**. A healthy esophagus is capable to handle occasional gastric refluxes through frequent peristalsis and the neutralization of salivary bicarbonate. However, due to various pathologic reasons, the esophageal motility becomes weak and consequently, the acidic refluxate cannot be cleared from the esophageal lumen instantly, resulting in mucosal damage and GERD symptoms. According to multiple studies, up to 63.95% of GERD patients were noted to have impaired esophageal peristalsis [14–16].

5. **Non-biological factors**. Several social economic factors have been repeatedly found in connection to GERD occurrence. For instance, people with an advanced degree of education are less likely to develop GERD [9]. The ratio is about 2:1 between the people who did not go to college (16.78%) and the ones who went beyond college education (8.98%). Marital status is also a factor. Singles (12.85%) are less likely to develop GERD than married, devoiced, or widowed individuals (22.95%). More interestingly, GERD is found more prevalent in developed countries than in developing or poor countries, but more common in people with low income (blue collars) than those in a better economic condition (white collars) [17]. The mechanisms behind all these observations are unclear.

Other controversial factors are noted in GERD development, including delayed gastric emptying, gastric acid over-secretion, age, gender, and race. Take gastric emptying as an example. For a normal person, the entire process from ingestion to defecation takes about 2–5 days to finish. After a meal, the stomach first relaxes to accommodate the ingested food and then breaks it down by rhythmic churning and grinding motions accompanied by the secretion of acid and digestive enzymes, which takes about 2–4 hours before releasing the food remnants into the small intestine for full digestion and absorption. Several factors can slow down the process, such as overeating, high-fat meals, low hormone secretion, low physical activity, and gastroparesis. In such cases, the accumulating food in the stomach builds up the intra-gastric pressure to push the gastroesophageal barrier to open, allowing the stomach contents to run into the esophagus instead of going down into the intestine [18, 19]. However, several studies did not find a strong correlation between delayed gastric emptying and GERD occurrence [20–22]. For this reason, using prokinetics to improve gastric motility is not recommended by American College of Gastroenterology (ACG) for GERD relief. Similarly, there are conflicting data about age. Biologically speaking, the gastroesophageal barrier should be like any other part of the body, growing stronger before 40 and getting weaker as the age approaches seniors. However, according to the meta-analysis [9], GERD is found in 8.70% of the people at the age of 18–34 and 14.53% in the age group of 35–59 but comes down after the age of 60.

4. How to cure GERD? we do not know

Because we cannot nail the ultimate cause of GERD, our treatment strategy for this disease is not targeted specifically. It involves changing eating habits, modifying lifestyle, suppressing gastric acid, and surgical intervention.

1. Changing eating habits

   As discussed above, many common foods and drinks have been found to trigger GERD occurrence, including coffee, tea, soda, juice, wine, liquor, chocolate, tomatoes, spicy food, high-fat food, etc. The question is can we really stop all of these?

2. Modifying lifestyle

   Compared to changing eating habits, modifying a lifestyle may be more doable. We can cut back on tobacco smoking or replace it with nicotine-free cigarettes. We can cut back on night snacks or avoid eating anything 3 hours before bed. We can sit straight during and after meals or stay up an hour or two after a meal. We can cut back the size of each meal to control the body weight. We can raise the head end of the bed or put one more pillow under the head before sleep. We can try to sleep on the left side more often. For some of us, this might be still a little hard to put into action, but we can always make effort for the sake of health.

3. Suppressing stomach acid

   It is commonly thought that acid is the main trigger for GERD symptoms. For this reason, tremendous effort has been put into developing anti-acid drugs. From anti-acids to H2 blockers (famotidine and cimetidine) to PPIs (omeprazole, lansoprazole, esomeprazole, pantoprazole, dexlansoprazole, and rabeprazole), it has been a multibillion industry that keeps growing year after year. Based on numerous studies, it is true that taking these drugs improves GERD symptoms effectively [23–25]. However, improving is not curing. The reduction of acid secretion is simply not enough to stop GERD completely. Increasing evidence suggests that acid reflux may contribute to esophageal erosion but does not lead to malignancy; it is the bile reflux that induces the development of Barrett's esophagus and adenocarcinoma [26–31].

4. Surgical intervention

Surgical intervention is the last option if other therapeutic management fails to achieve satisfaction. Among several GERD surgeries, laparoscopic Nissen fundoplication has been the gold standard, because it intends to restore the function of the gastroesophageal barrier [32]. However, patients undergoing fundoplication are at risk for developing postoperative adverse events, such as bloating, dysphagia, and belching. One study showed that 62% of the GERD patients who had fundoplication surgery came back on PPI medication later [33]. Magnetic sphincter augmentation (MSA) can be an alternative procedure to replace fundoplication. MSA uses a necklace of titanium beads with magnetic cores that encircle the distal esophagus and thereby strengthen the LES function. Compared with fundoplication, MSA is less invasive, and has a shorter operation time, less gas bloat, and better ability to belch and vomit [34]. For obesity-related GERD patients, Roux-en-Y gastric bypass (RYGB) is recommended by the ACG to be the best option [35–37]. However, a Swedish cohort study reported that among 2454 participants who had undergone RYGB, 48.8% (95% CI, 46.8–51.0) had GERD recurrence within 2 years of the operation [38].

5. Closing remarks

Despite the long history of GERD study and the tremendous effort that has been put in to find a cure, we still do not have the exact knowledge of how many people are affected, what causes the disease, and how to prevent the disease. Current treatment strategies simply cannot cure the disease. Maybe it is time to reexamine the evidence, come up with a different explanation, and explore the matter in a new direction.

Author details

Xianmei Meng and Jianyuan Chai*
Inner Mongolia Institute of Digestive Diseases, The Second Affiliated Hospital of Baotou Medical College, Inner Mongolia University of Science and Technology, Baotou, China

*Address all correspondence to: jianyuan.chai@gmail.com

References

[1] European Digestive Health Summit. Combatting the burden of digestive diseases through tighter controls on the alcohol and food industry. United European Gastroenterology Journal. 2018;**6**:159

[2] Brook RA, Wahlqvist P, Kleinman NL, Wallander MA, Campbell SM, Smeeding JE. Cost of gastro-oesophageal reflux disease to the employer: A perspective from the United States. Alimentary Pharmacology & Therapeutics. 2007;**26**(6):889-898. DOI: 10.1111/j.1365-2036.2007.03428.x

[3] Zagari RM, Fuccio L, Wallander MA, Johansson S, Fiocca R, Casanova S, et al. Gastro-oesophageal reflux symptoms, oesophagitis and Barrett's oesophagus in the general population: The Loiano-Monghidoro study. Gut. 2008;**57**(10):1354-1359. DOI: 10.1136/gut.2007.145177

[4] Dent J, Vakil N, Jones R, Bytzer P, Schöning U, Halling K, et al. Accuracy of the diagnosis of GORD by questionnaire, physicians and a trial of proton pump inhibitor treatment: The diamond study. Gut. 2010;**59**(6):714-721. DOI: 10.1136/gut.2009.200063

[5] Spechler SJ, Genta RM, Souza RF. Thoughts on the complex relationship between gastroesophageal reflux disease and eosinophilic esophagitis. The American Journal of Gastroenterology. 2007;**102**:1301-1306

[6] Tack J, Caenepeel P, Arts J, Lee KJ, Sifrim D, Janssens J. Prevalence of acid reflux in functional dyspepsia and its association with symptom profile. Gut. 2005;**54**(10):1370-1376. DOI: 10.1136/gut.2004.053355

[7] Gourcerol G, Benanni Y, Boueyre E, Leroi AM, Ducrotte P. Influence of gastric emptying on gastro-esophageal reflux: A combined pH-impedance study. Neurogastroenterology and Motility. 2013;**25**(10):800-e634. DOI: 10.1111/nmo.12181

[8] Vakil N, van Zanten SV, Kahrilas P, Dent J, Jones R. Global Consensus Group. The Montreal definition and classification of gastroesophageal reflux disease: A global evidence-based consensus. The American Journal of Gastroenterology. 2006;**101**(8):1900-1920. DOI: 10.1111/j.1572-0241.2006.00630.x

[9] Nirwan JS, Hasan SS, Babar Z, Conway BR, Ghori MU. Global prevalence and risk factors of gastro-oesophageal reflux disease (GORD): Systematic review with meta-analysis. Scientific Reports. 2020;**10**:5814. DOI: 10.1038/s41598-020-62795-1

[10] Fuchs KH, Lee AM, Breithaupt W, Varga G, Babic B, Horgan S. Pathophysiology of gastroesophageal reflux disease – Which factors are important? Translational Gastroenterology and Hepatology. 2021;**6**:53. DOI: 10.21037/tgh.2020.02.12

[11] Eusebi LH, Ratnakumaran R, Yuan Y, Solaymani-Dodaran M, Bazzoli F, Ford AC. Global prevalence of, and risk factors for, gastro-oesophageal reflux symptoms: A meta-analysis. Gut. 2018;**67**(3):430-440

[12] De Giorgi F, Palmiero M, Esposito I, Mosca F, Cuomo R. Pathophysiology of gastro-oesophageal reflux disease. Acta Otorhinolaryngologica Italica. 2006;**26**(5):241-246

[13] Mittal RK, McCallum RW. Characteristics and frequency of transient relaxations of the lower esophageal sphincter in patients with reflux esophagitis. Gastroenterology. 1988;**95**(3):593-599

[14] Diener U, Patti MG, Molena D, Fisichella PM, Way LW. Esophageal dysmotility and gastroesophageal reflux disease. Journal of Gastrointestinal Surgery. 2001;**5**(3):260-265

[15] Shetler KP, Bikhtii S, Triadafilopoulos G. Ineffective esophageal motility: Clinical, manometric, and outcome characteristics in patients with and without abnormal esophageal acid exposure. Diseases of the Esophagus. 2017;**30**:1-8

[16] Jiang LQ, Ye BX, Wang MF, Lin L. Acid exposure in patients with gastroesophageal reflux disease is associated with esophageal dysmotility. Journal of Digestive Diseases. 2019;**20**:73-77

[17] Zheng Z, Shang Y, Wang N, Liu X, Xin C, Yan X, et al. Current advancement on the dynamic mechanism of gastroesophageal reflux disease. International Journal of Biological Sciences. 2021;**17**:4154-4164. DOI: 10.7150/ijbs.65066

[18] Penagini R, Bravi I. The role of delayed gastric emptying and impaired oesophageal body motility. Best Practice & Research. Clinical Gastroenterology. 2010;**24**:831-845

[19] Richter JE, Rubenstein JH. Presentation and epidemiology of gastroesophageal reflux disease. Gastroenterology. 2018;**154**:267-276

[20] Camlleri M, Parkman HP, Shafi MA, Abell TL, Gerson L. Clinical guideline: Management of gastroparesis. The American Journal of Gastroenterology. 2013;**108**:18-37

[21] Gourcel G, Benanni Y, Boueyre E, Leroi AM, Ducrotte P. Influence of gastric emptying on gastroesophageal reflux: A combined pH-impedance study. Neurogastroenterology and Motility. 2013;**25**:800-807

[22] Stacher G, Lenglinger J, Bergmann H, Schneider C, Hoffmann M, Wolfl G, et al. Gastric emptying: A contributory factor in gastro-oesophageal reflux activity? Gut. 2000;**47**:661-666

[23] Zhang JX, Ji MY, Song J, Lei HB, Qiu S, Wang J, et al. Proton pump inhibitor for non-erosive reflux disease: A meta-analysis. World Journal of Gastroenterology. 2013;**19**(45):8408-8419

[24] Robinson M, Sahba B, Avner D, Jhala N, Greski-Rose PA, Jennings DE. A comparison of lansoprazole and ranitidine in the treatment of erosive oesophagitis. Multicentre Investigational Group. Alimentary Pharmacology and Therapeutics. 1995;**9**(1):25-31. DOI: 10.1111/j.1365-2036.1995.tb00347.x

[25] Kirchheiner J, Glatt S, Fuhr U, Klotz U, Meineke I, Seufferlein T, et al. Relative potency of proton-pump inhibitors-comparison of effects on intragastric pH. European Journal of Clinical Pharmacology. 2009;**65**(1):19-31. DOI: 10.1007/s00228-008-0576-5

[26] Souza RF. The role of acid and bile reflux in esophagitis and Barrett's metaplasia. Biochemical Society Transactions. 2010;**38**:348-352

[27] Debruyne PR, Witek M, Gong L, Birbe R, Chervoneva I, Jin T, et al. Bile acids induce ectopic expression of intestinal guanylyl cyclase through

nuclear factor-κB and CDX2 in human esophageal cells. Gastroenterology. 2006;**130**:1191-1206

[28] Chai J. Esophagus and esophageal cancer. In: Chai J, editor. Esophageal Cancer and beyond. London: IntechOpen; 2018. pp. 1-10. DOI: 10.5772/intechopen.77995

[29] Dang T, Meng X, Modak C, Wu J, Chang Z, Che N, et al. Overexpression of CCN1 in Het1A cells attenuates bile-induced esophageal metaplasia through suppressing non-canonical NFκB activation. Cytokine. 2019;**116**:61-69. DOI: 10.1016/j.cyto.2018.12.020

[30] Dang T, Chai J. Molecular dynamics in Esophageal adenocarcinoma: Who's in control? Current Cancer Drug Targets. 2020;**20**:789-801. DOI: 10.2174/1568009620666200720011341

[31] Chang Z, Dang T, Meng X, Chai J. The role of CCN1 in Esophageal adenocarcinoma: What we have learned from the lab. Cancer Control. 2022;**29**(1-9):10732748221074734. DOI: 10.1177/10732748221074734

[32] Spechler SJ, Lee E, Ahnen D, Goyal RK, Hirano I, Ramirez F, et al. Long-term outcome of medical and surgical therapies for gastroesophageal reflux disease: Follow-up of a randomized controlled trial. Journal of the American Medical Association. 2001;**285**(18):2331-2338. DOI: 10.1001/jama.285.18.2331

[33] Maret-Ouda J, Wahlin K, El-Serag HB, Lagergren J. Association between laparoscopic antireflux surgery and recurrence of gastroesophageal reflux. Journal of the American Medical Association. 2017;**318**(10):939-946. DOI: 10.1001/jama.2017.10981

[34] Aiolfi A, Asti E, Bernardi D, Bonitta G, Rausa E, Siboni S, et al. Early results of magnetic sphincter augmentation versus fundoplication for gastroesophageal reflux disease: Systematic review and meta-analysis. International Journal of Surgery. 2018;**52**:82-88. DOI: 10.1016/j.ijsu.2018.02.041

[35] Katz PO, Dunbar KB, Schnoll-Sussman FH, Greer KB, Yadlapati R, Jon SS. ACG Clinical Guideline for the diagnosis and management of gastroesophageal reflux disease. The American Journal of Gastroenterology. 2022;**117**:27-56. DOI: 10.14309/ajg.0000000000001538

[36] Sandhu DS, Fass R. Current trends in the Management of Gastroesophageal Reflux Disease. Gut Liver. 2018;**12**(1):7-16

[37] Chang P, Friedenberg F. Obesity and GERD. Gastroenterology Clinics of North America. 2014;**43**(1):161-173

[38] Holmberg D, Santoni G, Xie S, Lagergren J. Gastric bypass surgery in the treatment of gastro-oesophageal reflux symptoms. Alimentary Pharmacology & Therapeutics. 2019;**50**(2):159-166. DOI: 10.1111/apt.15274

Chapter 2

Gastroesophageal Reflux Disease and Obesity

I Dewa Nyoman Wibawa and Ni Wayan Wina Dharmesti

Abstract

The global rise of gastroesophageal reflux disease (GERD) prevalence makes it one of the most common diagnoses performed in a daily practice. Obesity significantly contribute to GERD development, accordingly, it has accounted for the increasing cases of GERD. Obesity can disrupt the esophagogastric junction integrity, which promote the development of GERD and its complication. The frequency of GERD symptoms and its mucosal complications also found more often in obesity. The parallel increase of both condition has initiated numerous studies to determine the most beneficial therapeutic options in managing this challenging condition. Current available therapy for GERD in obesity including weight reduction, pharmacotherapy, and surgery.

Keywords: GERD, obesity, erosive esophagitis, treatment, pathophysiology of GERD, GERD management

1. Introduction

Occasional reflux of gastric content into the esophagus is a physiological phenomenon, until it presents with symptoms and/or mucosal complication, which defines the condition of GERD [1]. GERD is one of the most common diagnoses performed in a daily practice [2]. Clinically, GERD may manifest with cardinal symptoms of heartburn and regurgitation. Other symptoms are classified as esophageal (e.g., dysphagia, chest pain) and extraesophageal (atypical) symptoms [3]. GERD encompassed several subgroups, based on endoscopy and histopathological findings, such as erosive esophagitis, Barrett's esophagus, and nonerosive reflux disease (NERD) [3].

Recent evidence showed a rising prevalence of GERD and it was estimated 1.03 billion individuals are suffering from GERD globally [4, 5]. GERD has also become more prevalent nowadays in a previously uncommon region, such as Asia Pacific [6]. Excessive body weight is one of the multiple conditions that contribute to this escalation in GERD cases [7]. Yamasaki *et al.* in their study discovered a characteristic finding of GERD patients were primarily obese or severely obese [7]. Many of previous studies showed a common finding of reflux symptoms in patients with obesity, indicated an association between GERD and obesity [8]. The risk of both reflux symptoms and mucosal injury related to GERD is found to be increased in obesity [9]. Metabolic syndrome also appears to play a role in the development of GERD, since it independently increased the probability of NERD progression into erosive esophagitis [10]. Given the background of growing burden in both conditions, the following sections will discuss the pathophysiology and available therapeutic modalities for GERD in obese individuals.

2. GERD in obesity

Obesity has reached an epidemic proportion globally [11]. This condition is diagnosed when the measured body mass index (BMI) is ≥30 kg/m^2 and further classified into three group based on its severity levels: class I (BMI 30.0–34.9), class II (BMI 35.0–39.9), and class III (BMI ≥40.0) [11]. Epidemiological study have shown that obesity is a major risk factor for GERD and, consequently, has accounted for the increasing prevalence of GERD, worldwide [12]. Study by Hampel *et al.* showed overweight and obesity fulfill a number criteria for a causal relationship with GERD [9]. Previous studies also discovered the influence of BMI on GERD was not affected by nutritional intake [13–15].

Study by Murray *et al.* showed that subjects with obesity reported more frequent heartburn compared to the subjects with normal weight (OR 2.91) and this obese subjects also showed significant association with severe heartburn (OR 1.19) [13]. A dose–response relationship between frequency of heartburn or regurgitation and high BMI was observed by El-Serag *et al.* [16]. This study also found subjects with mucosal erosion were more often to be overweight or obese, compared to subjects without erosion [16].

2.1 Pathophysiology of GERD in obesity

Since obesity has contributed largely to the increased of GERD prevalence, there has been a substantial attention to explore the possible mechanisms of GERD development in obesity [17]. The essential pathology in the development of GERD is excessive acid and bile salt exposure on the gastric mucosa [3]. This abnormal exposure may lead to distressing symptoms of GERD when the number of reflux events is enormous, the period of mucosal exposure to gastric content is prolonged, there is concomitant defect in mucosal integrity, or hypersensitivity to refluxate [3]. The integrity of the esophagogastric junction (EGJ), both structural and functional, is an important antireflux barrier [3]. Major mechanisms of EGJ incompetence that discovered in GERD are anatomical derangement of the EGJ including hiatal hernia, decreased pressure of lower esophageal sphincter (LES), and transient lower esophageal sphincter relaxation (TLESR). Delayed gastric emptying and prolonged esophageal clearance time has been found in subsets of patients as mechanism that may exacerbate GERD [3].

Several factors that could increase acid exposure time on the esophagus was found more often in patients with obesity than in individuals with normal weight [12]. The development of GERD in obese individuals was previously thought to be mainly structural, owing to the weight of abdominal fat that increase intra-abdominal pressure, thereby increased the likelihood reflux occurrence. Recent evidence also suggest that obesity may alter the physiologic function of lower esophageal sphincter (decreased LES pressure, increased frequency of transient LES relaxation), and/or gastroesophageal motility (delayed esophageal clearing time, impaired gastric emptying) [9, 13].

The development of a hiatal hernia is the main factor that disrupts the integrity of the EGJ in patients with excess body weight [9]. The prevalence of hiatal hernia is significantly higher in subjects with obesity than in subjects with a normal BMI [18]. The physiological explanation for the interplay between obesity, risk for hiatal hernia, and subsequent development of GERD was thoroughly explored in a manometry study conducted by Pandolfino *et al* [19]. Their study discovered an altered pressure morphology within and across the EGJ in obese subjects that would augment the movement of acid and bile salts toward the esophagus. Obesity caused greater axial separation between the LES and the diaphragm, that ultimately lead to the development of hiatal hernia [19]. This proximal displacement of the LES creates a lower basal pressure of LES, diminishes the increment in LES pressure that occurs during straining, and increases transient LES relaxation (TLESR) frequency during gastric distention with gas [20, 21]. Transient LES relaxation seems to be the most important mechanism responsible for reflux [22]. Overweight and obese patients showed a significantly higher TLESR rate during the post-prandial period as compared to subjects with normal BMI [23]. It also appeared that both BMI and waist circumference have a dose-effect relationship with TLESR [23].

Central obesity also play a part in the pathogenesis of GERD [18]. Current data suggest that central obesity causes an increase in intra-gastric pressure, which subsequently increased esophageal exposure to gastric content and impaired esophageal acid clearance [24, 25]. Moreover, the visceral fat is a metabolically active organ that produces interleukin-6 and tumor necrosis factor-α, that may have impact on LES. Recent data also suggest that insulin resistance, a consequence of visceral obesity, may be an important contributing factor [26]. Studies also found that abdominal obesity may change the secretion of adipokines such as adiponectin and leptin that has been regarded as the key factor for the development of esophageal neoplasia in the setting of obesity [12, 17]. Adipokine has anti-inflammatory and immunomodulatory properties and may stimulate apoptosis [27]. Obesity decrease the secretion of adiponectin and this was associated with increased risk of BE [28]. Leptin has been shown to have mitogenic properties, that later study found it may induce proliferation of esophageal cancer [29]. Kendall *et al.* found the risk of BE were higher in subjects with high level of serum leptin (OR 4.6) [30]. All of the proposed mechanisms that promotes the development of GERD in obesity is summarized in **Figure 1**.

The traditional theory of refluxed gastric content has caused direct injury to the esophageal mucosa, as discussed above, is challenged by the findings of recent studies in rats and human that found the exposure of esophageal mucosa to gastric content did not cause a direct acid injury in the esophagus [31, 32]. Instead, it stimulated the esophageal mucosa to secrete cytokines that induce proliferative changes in epithelial cells and attract the T lymphocyte and other pro-inflammatory cells that eventually caused mucosal damage [31, 32]. Hypoxia-inducible factor-2α (HIF-2α) is a transcription factor that is involved in the mediation of some inflammatory response [33] and appear to be the key mediator that initiate the cytokine-mediated mucosal injury [34]. The exposure gastric juice to esophageal epithelial cells leads to the production of reactive oxygen species, a key substance to stabilize HIF-2α in the setting of GERD [35, 36]. This stabilized HIF-2α will accumulate in the nucleus and stimulate the secretion of inflammatory cytokines that lead to the establishment of GERD [34]. This new paradigm in GERD pathogenesis, however, has not been studied in term of its possible role in GERD with obesity. Nonetheless, this undisclosed association between cytokine-mediated mucosal injury and obesity in the pathogenesis of GERD may serve as an opportunity for researches in the future.

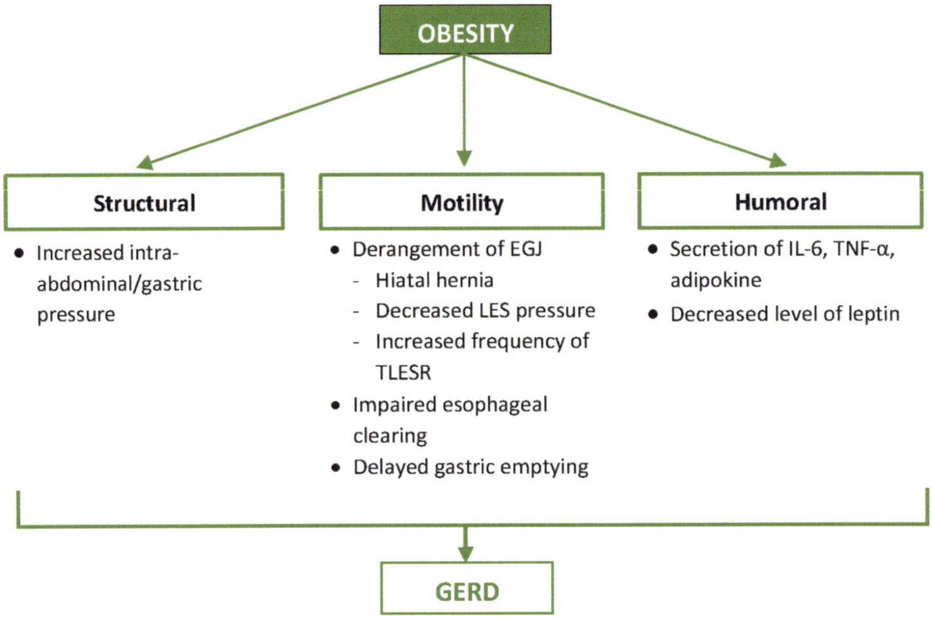

Figure 1.
Pathophysiology of GERD in obesity. EGJ, esophagogastric junction; GERD, gastroesophageal reflux disease; IL-6, interleukin-6; TNF-α, tumor necrosis factor-α; LES, lower esophageal sphincter; TLESR, transient lower esophageal sphincter relaxation.

3. Management

Management of GERD requires more than one approach, which considered the symptom severity, endoscopic findings, and possible physiological abnormalities [36]. Treatment modalities includes lifestyle modification, pharmacologic therapy, and surgery [36]. The growing attention to the reflux problems in patients with obesity has prompted a numerous studies to obtain the most beneficial therapeutic options [18]. In the following section, recent evidences that support the beneficial effect of particular treatment options in GERD patients with obesity will be discussed.

3.1 Weight reduction

Lifestyle modification is the recommended first step in the treatment of GERD. However, the only measures that have been shown to be beneficial on the part of obese patient is weight loss [37]. Weight loss is strongly recommended in overweight or obese GERD patients to improve the reflux symptoms [6, 36]. A prospective cohort study has found that in GERD subjects with overweight and obesity, weight reduction was significantly decreased the overall prevalence of GERD with significant improvement in overall symptoms scoring, compared to baseline [38]. The result of this study also showed a substantial reduction in overall GERD scores only observed among subjects who loss body weight ≥5% from baseline. Study conducted by de Bortoli *et al*. found that group of GERD patients who had weight reduction was showing not only a higher rate of symptoms improvement, but also managed to reduce the dosage of proton pump inhibitor (PPI), compared to group without weight reduction [39].

This study also recommend all patients with GERD to achieve a minimum 10% weight loss from baseline in order to hasten the efficacy of PPI to relieve GERD symptom [39]. The result of the above studies is supported by the finding of dose-dependent relationship between reduction in body weight and improvement of GERD symptoms [40]. Study conducted by Park *et al* found weight reduction was significantly associated with improvement of GERD symptom, but showed no association with improvement in erosive esophagitis [41].

3.2 Pharmacotherapy

PPI are the mainstay medical treatment for GERD, it is initially given as active-phase therapy, with continuous use to improve and heal the mucosal erosion, then follows by on-demand therapy phase for maintenance [6, 36]. However, there are still scarce yet inconsistent data available regarding the influence of obesity to the response of PPI treatment for GERD patients. Peura *et al.* conducted a study that found the efficacy of PPI therapy on the reduction in heartburn symptoms frequency and severity was similar across BMI categories, in both NERD and erosive esophagitis patients [42]. However, when the therapeutic target of the initial phase of PPI therapy is based on the sustained symptomatic response (SSR, *i.e.* free from reflux symptoms for the last 7 days), Sheu *et al.* found a lower SSR rates in the overweight and obese groups, compared to control group [43]. During maintenance therapy, the mean number of PPI tablets used was significantly higher in the overweight and obese groups than in the control group [43]. This findings was further studied by Chen *et al.* to determine whether double-dose PPI can elevate the SSR rate for overweight or obese patients [44]. They also checked whether different genotypes of CYP2C19 would affect the SSR rates. This study found a higher rates of SSR in the double-dose PPI group than in the standard group. Treatment with double-dosed PPI also improved the cumulative rates of SSR in the extensive metabolizer group [44].

Pharmacotherapy in obesity is indicated in patients with obesity-associated complications that have failed to achieve a healthy weight by implementing a low-calorie diet and regular exercise [45]. Less coverage of antiobesity drugs by insurance and their high cost has limits patients' choices. In addition, until the present time there is no available data that describe the impact of using antiobesity to achieve weight loss in patients with GERD.

3.3 Surgery

Antireflux surgery is an alternative for long-term treatment of GERD patients with severe reflux esophagitis (LA grade C or D), large hiatal hernias, and/or persistent distressing GERD symptoms [36]. Laparoscopic antireflux surgery (Nissen fundoplication, Toupet fundoplication) has been viewed as an alternative to lifelong PPI treatment in GERD [18]. The efficacy and safety of this procedure in patient with obesity, however is still controversial [46, 47]. Therefore bariatric surgery (Roux-en-Y gastric bypass) is being more considered recently as a procedure of choice for GERD in patient with morbid obesity [18]. Bariatric surgery was able to achieve substantial weight reduction and lower abdominal-thoracic pressure gradient [18]. Many studies have shown consistent improvement in both reflux symptoms and mucosal complication of GERD following a bariatric procedure in obese patients [18]. Nonetheless, it must be highlighted that all patients, require a lifelong and multidisciplinary follow up care after bariatric surgery [18].

Laparoscopic sleeve gastrectomy (LSG) is another approach of bariatric procedure that has gained more attention, owing to less technical complexity as compare to laparoscopic Roux-en-Y gastric bypass (LRYGB), it showed lower incidence of postoperative complication, and leads to substantial weight loss [48]. The impact of LSG on GERD, however is still inconsistent in regards to the control of pre-existing reflux, development of *de novo* GERD after procedure, and several studies suggested that LSG is a refluxogenic procedure [49–51]. Another study showed that the main technical issues that determine the occurrence of postoperative GERD are relative narrowing of the sleeve and hiatal hernia [52]. Ultimately, the baseline severity of reflux symptoms and mucosal injury is the key determinants of patient's feasibility to surgery [51]. Erosive esophagitis is considered as a relative contraindication to the surgery by the joint statement of ASMBS, SAGES, and ASGE [53]. Recently, the available management options for GERD after LSG include pharmacotherapy with PPI or repair with laparoscopic Roux-en-Y gastric bypass [52]. These available options should be openly discussed with the patients [51].

4. Conclusions

Obesity is a major risk factor of GERD and has accounted for the rising GERD case, worldwide. The fundamental mechanisms in the development of GERD were found more frequently in patients with obesity. Accordingly, the frequency of reflux symptoms and mucosal complications of GERD were also higher in obese patients. Current available treatment options has highlight the benefit of weight loss in GERD patients with obesity, not only to improve the symptoms but also to enhance the response to GERD pharmacotherapy. Role of antiobesity pharmacotherapy is still limited in GERD patients. Those patients who failed the conservative medical therapy may be considered for surgical procedure to achieve weight reduction and improvement of GERD symptoms. The baseline reflux symptoms severity and mucosal injury are key factors in determining which patients that will benefit from surgery. The possible postoperative complication and available management options should be openly discussed with patients.

Acknowledgements

No financial support was received for this work.

Conflict of interest

The authors declare no conflict of interest.

Author details

I Dewa Nyoman Wibawa* and Ni Wayan Wina Dharmesti
Division of Gastroentero-Hepatology, Internal Medicine Department, Medical Faculty of Udayana University, Sanglah Hospital, Bali, Indonesia

*Address all correspondence to: dnwib@dps.centrin.net.id

References

[1] Vakil N, van Zanten SV, Kahrilas P, Dent J, Jones R, Global Consensus Group. Montreal definition and classification of gastroesophageal reflux disease: A global evidence-based consensus. The American Journal of Gastroenterology. 2006;**101**(8):1900-1920. DOI: 10.1111/j.1572-0241.2006.00630.x

[2] Katzka DA, Pandolfino JE, Kahrilas PJ. Phenotypes of gastroesophageal reflux diseases: Where Rome, Lyon, and Montreal meet. Clinical Gastroenterology and Hepatology. 2020;**18**:767-776. DOI: 10.1016/j.cgh.2019.07.015

[3] Roman S, Pandolfino JE, Kahrilas PJ. Gastroesophageal reflux disease. In: Podolsky DK, Camilleri M, Fitz JG, Kalloo AN, Shanahan F, Wang TC, editors. Yamada's Textbook of Gastroenterology. Sixth ed. Oxford: John Wiley & Sons; 2016. pp. 906-928

[4] Boulton KHA, Dettmar PW. A narrative review of the prevalence of gastroesophageal reflux disease (GERD). Annals of Esophagus. 2022;**5**:7. DOI: 10.21037/aoe-20-80

[5] Nirwan JS, Hasan SS, Babar ZUD, Conway BR, Ghori MU. Global prevalence and risk factors of gastro-esophageal reflux disease (GORD): Systematic review with meta-analysis. Scientific Reports. 2020;**10**:5814. DOI: 10.1038/s41598-020-62795-1

[6] Goh KL, Lee YY, Leelakusolvong S, Makmun D, Maneerattanaporn M, Quach DT, et al. Consensus statement and recommendations on the management of mild-to-moderate gastroesophageal reflux disease in the southeast Asian region. JGH Open. 2021;**5**:855-863. DOI: 10.1002/jgh3.12602

[7] Yamasaki T, Hemond C, Eisa M, Ganocy S, Fass R. The changing epidemiology of GERD: Are patients getting younger. Journal of Neurogastroenterology and Motility. 2018;**24**(4):559-569. DOI: 10.5056/jnm18140

[8] El-Serag H. The association between obesity and GERD: A review of the epidemiological evidence. Digestive Diseases and Sciences. 2008;**53**(9):2307-2312. DOI: 10.1007/s10620-008-0413-9

[9] Hampel H, Abraham NS, El-Serag HB. Meta-analysis: Obesity and the risk for gastroesophageal reflux disease and its complications. Annals of Internal Medicine. 2005;**143**:199-211. DOI: 10.7326/0003-4819-143-3-200508020-00006

[10] Hershcovici T, Fass R. Nonerosive reflux disease (NERD)-an update. Journal of Neurogastroenterology and Motility. 2010;**16**(1):8-21. DOI: 10.5056/jnm.2010.16.18

[11] Haththotuwa RN, Wijeyaratne CN, Senarath U. Worldwide epidemic of obesity. In: Mahmood TA, Chervenak FA, Arulkumaran S, editors. Obesity and Obstetrics Second ed. Amsterdam: Elsevier; 2020. pp. 3-8. DOI: 10.1016/C201-8-0-02230-6

[12] Chang P, Friedenberg F. Obesity & GERD. Gastroenterology Clinics of North America. 2014;**43**(1):161-173. DOI: 10.1016/j.gtc.2013.11.009

[13] Murray L, Johnston B, Lane A, Harvey I, Donovan J, Nair P, et al. Relationship between body mass index and gastro-esophageal reflux symptoms: The Bristol Helicobacter project. International Journal of Epidemiology. 2003;**32**:645-650. DOI: 10.1093/ije/dyg108

[14] Nilsson M, Johnsen R, Ye W, Hveem K, Lagergren J. Obesity and estrogen as risk factors for gastroesophageal reflux symptoms. Journal of the American Medical Association. 2003;**290**:66-72. DOI: 10.1001/jama.290.1.66

[15] Nandurkar S, Locke GR 3rd, Fett S, Zinsmeister AR, Cameron AJ, Talley AJ. Relationship between body mass index, diet, exercise, and gastro-esophageal reflux symptoms in community. Alimentary Pharmacology & Therapeutics. 2004;**20**:497-505. DOI: 10.1111/j.1365-2036.2004.02156.x

[16] El-Serag HB, Graham DY, Satia JA, Rabeneck L. Obesity is an independent risk factor for GERD symptoms and erosive esophagitis. The American Journal of Gastroenterology. 2005;**100**(6):1243-1250. DOI: 10.1111/j.1572-0241.2005.41703.x

[17] Emerenziani S, Rescio MP, Guarino MPL, Cicala M. Gastro-esophageal reflux disease and obesity, where is the link? World Journal of Gastroenterology. 2013;**19**(39):6536-6539. DOI: 10.3748/wjg.v19.i39.6536

[18] Thalheimer A, Bueter M. Excess of body weight and gastroesophageal reflux disease. Visceral Medicine. 2021;**37**:267-272. DOI: 10.1159/000516050

[19] Pandolfino JE, El-Serag HB, Zhang Q, Shah N, Ghosh SK, Kahrilas PJ. Obesity: A challenge to esophagogastric junction integrity. Gastroenterology. 2006;**130**:639-649. DOI: 10.1053/j.gastro.2005.12.016

[20] Mattioli S, D'Ovidio F, Pilotti V, Di Simone MP, Lugaresi M, Bassi F, et al. Hiatus hernia and intrathoracic migration of the esophagogastric junction in gastroesophageal reflux disease. Digestive Diseases and Sciences. 2003;**48**:1823-1831. DOI: 10.1023/A:1025471801571

[21] Kahrilas P, Shi G, Manka M, Joehll R. Increased frequency of transient lower esophageal sphincter relaxation induced by gastric distention in reflux patients with hiatal hernia. Gastroenterology. 2000;**118**:688-695. DOI: 10.1016/S0016-5085(00)70138-7

[22] Sifrim D, Holloway R. Transient lower esophageal sphincter relaxations: How many or how harmful? The American Journal of Gastroenterology. 2001;**96**:2529-2532. DOI: 10.1111/j.1572-0241.2001.04095

[23] Wu JC, Mui LM, Cheung CM, Chan Y, Sung JJ. Obesity is associated with increased transient lower esophageal sphincter relaxation. Gastroenterology. 2007;**132**:883-889. DOI: 10.1053/j.gastro.2006.12.032

[24] Derakhsan MH, Robertson EV, Fletcher J, Jones GR, Lee YY, Wirz AA, et al. Mechanism of association between BMI and dysfunction of the gastro-esophageal barrier in patients with normal endoscopy. Gut. 2012;**61**(3):337-343. DOI: 10.1136/gutjnl-2011-300633

[25] Ringhofer C, Lengliner J, Riegler M, Kristo I, Kainz A, Schoppmann SF. Waist to hip ratio is a better predictor of esophageal acid exposure than body mass index. Neurogastroenterology and Motility. 2017;**29**(7):e13033. DOI: 10.1111/nmo.13033

[26] Hsu CS, Wang PC, Chen JH. Increasing insulin resistance is associated with increased severity and prevalence of gastro-esophageal reflux disease. Alimentary Pharmacology & Therapeutics. 2011;**34**:994-1004. DOI: 10.1111/j.1365-2036.2011.04817.x

[27] Kelesidis I, Kelesidis T, Mantzoros CS. Adiponectin and cancer: A systematic review. British Journal of Cancer. 2006;**94**(9):1221-1225. DOI: 10.1038/sj.bjc.6603051

[28] Rubenstein JH, Kao JY, Madanick RD, Zhang M, Wang M, Spacek MB, et al. Association of adiponectin multimers with Barrett's oesophagus. Gut. 2009;**58**(12):1583-1589. DOI: 10.1136%2Fgut.2008.171553

[29] Ogunwobi O, Mutungi G, Beales IL. Leptin stimulates proliferation and inhibits apoptosis in Barrett's esophageal adenocarcinoma cells by cyclooxygenase-2-dependent, prostaglandin-E2-mediated transactivation of the epidermal growth factor receptor and c-Jun NH2-terminal kinase activation. Endocrinology. 2006;**147**(9):4505-4516. DOI: 10.1210/en.2006-0224

[30] Kendall BJ, Macdonald GA, Hayward NK, Prins JB, Brown I, Walker N, et al. Leptin and the risk of Barrett's oesophagus. Gut. 2008;**57**(4):448-454. DOI: 10.1136/gut.2007.131243

[31] Souza RF, Huo X, Mittal V, Schuler CM, Carmack SW, Zhang HY, et al. Gastroesophageal reflux might cause esophagitis through a cytokine-mediated mechanism rather than caustic acid injury. Gastroenterology. 2009;**137**:1776-1784. DOI: 10.1053/j.gastro.2009.07.055

[32] Dunbar KB, Agoston AT, Odze RD, Huo X, Pham TH, Cipher DJ, et al. Association of acute gastroesophageal reflux disease with esophageal histologic changes. Journal of the American Medical Association. 2016;**315**:2104-2112. DOI: 10.1001/jama.2016.5657

[33] Taylor CT. Interdependent roles for hypoxia inducible factor and nuclear factor-kappaB in hypoxic inflammation. The Journal of Physiology. 2008;**586**:4055-4059. DOI: 10.1113/jphysiol.2008.157669

[34] Souza RF, Bayeh L, Spechler SJ, Tambar UK, Bruick RK. A new paradigm for GERD pathogenesis: Not acid injury, but cytokine-mediated inflammation driven by HIF-2α: A potential role for targeting HIF-2α to prevent and treat reflux esophagitis. Current Opinion in Pharmacology. 2017;**37**:93-99. DOI: 10.1016/j.coph.2017.10.004

[35] Feagins LA, Zhang HY, Zhang X, Hormi-Carver K, Thomas T, Terada LS, et al. Mechanisms of oxidant production in esophageal squamous cell and Barrett's cell lines. American Journal of Physiology. Gastrointestinal and Liver Physiology. 2008;**294**:G411-G417. DOI: 10.1152/ajpgi.00373.207

[36] Katz PO, Dunbar KB, Schnoll-Sussman FH, Greer KB, Yadlapati R, Spechler SJ. ACG clinical guideline for the diagnosis and management of gastroesophageal reflux disease. The American Journal of Gastroenterology. 2022;**117**:27-56. DOI: 10.14309/ajg.0000000000001538

[37] Eherer A. Management of gastroesophageal reflux disease: Lifestyle modification and alternative approaches. Digestive Diseases. 2014;**32**:149-151. DOI: 10.1159%2F000357181

[38] Singh M, Lee J, Gupta N, Gaddam S, Smith BK, Wani SB, et al. Weight loss can lead to resolution of gastroesophageal reflux disease symptoms: A prospective interventional trial. Obesity (Silver Spring). 2013;**21**(2):284-290. DOI: 10.1002/oby.20279

[39] De Bortoli N, Guidi G, Martinucci I, Savarino E, Imam H, Bertani L, et al. Voluntary and controlled weight loss

can reduce symptoms and protom pump inhibitor use and dosage in patients with gastroesophageal reflux disease: A comparative study. Diseases of the Esophagus. 2014;**29**(2):197-204. DOI: 10.1111/dote.12319

[40] Ness-Jensen E, Lindam A, Lagergren J, Hveem K. Weight loss and reduction in gastroesophageal reflux. A prospective population-based cohort study: The HUNT study. The American Journal of Gastroenterology. 2013;**108**:376-382. DOI: 10.1038/ajg.2012.466

[41] Park SK, Lee T, Yang HJ, Park JH, Sohn CI, Ryu S, et al. Weight loss and waist reduction is associated with improvement in gastroesophageal disease reflux symptoms: A longitudinal study of 15295 subjects undergoing health checkups. Neurogastroenterology and Motility. 2016;**29**(5):1-7. DOI: 10.1111/nmo.13009

[42] Peura DA, Pilmer B, Hunt B, Mody R, Perez MC. The effects of increasing body mass index on heartburn severity, frequency and response to treatment with dexlansoprazole or lansoprazole. Alimentary Pharmacology & Therapeutics. 2013;**37**:810-818. DOI: 10.1111/apt.12270

[43] Sheu BS, Cheng HC, Chang WL, Chen WY, Kao AW. The impact of body mass index on the application of on-demand therapy for Los Angeles grades A and B reflux esophagitis. The American Journal of Gastroenterology. 2007;**102**:2387-2394. DOI: 10.1111/j.1572-0241.2007.01468.x

[44] Chen WY, Chang WL, Tsai YC, Cheng HC, Lu CC, Sheu BS. Double-dosed pantoprazole accelerates the sustained symptomatic response in overweight ang obese patients with reflux esophagitis in Los Angeles grade a and B. The American Journal of Gastroenterology. 2010;**105**(5):1046-1052. DOI: 10.138/ajg.2009.632

[45] Apovian CM, Aronne LJ, Bessenen DH, McDonnell ME, Murad MH, Pagotto U, et al. Pharmacological management of obesity: An endocrine society clinical practice guideline. The Journal of Clinical Endocrinology and Metabolism. 2015;**100**(2):342-362. DOI: 10.1210/jc.2014-3415

[46] Tekin K, Toydemir T, Yerdel MA. Is laparoscopic antireflux surgery safe and effective in obese patients? Surgical Endoscopy. 2012;**26**(1):86-95. DOI: 10.1007/s00464-011-1832-9

[47] Morgenthal CB, Lin E, Shane MD, Hunter JG, Smith CD. Who will fail laparoscopic Nissen fundoplication? Preoperative prediction of long-term outcomes. Surgical Endoscopy. 2007;**21**(11):1978-1984. DOI: 10.1007/s00464-007-9490-7

[48] Gadiot RP, Biter LU, van Mil S, Zengerink HF, Apers J, Mannaerts GH. Long-term results of laparoscopic sleeve gastrectomy for morbid obesity: 5 to 8-year results. Obesity Surgery. 2017;**27**:59-63. DOI: 10.1007/s11695-016-2235-8

[49] Oor JE, Roks DJ, Ünlü Ç, Hazebroek EJ. Laparoscopic sleeve gastrectomy and gastroesophageal reflux disease: A systematic review and meta-analysis. American Journal of Surgery. 2016;**211**:250-267. DOI: 10.1016/j.amjsurg.2015.05.031

[50] Mion F, Tolone S, Garros A, Savarino E, Pelascini E, Robert M, et al. High-resolution impedance manometry after sleeve gastrectomy: Increased intragastric pressure and reflux are frequent events. Obesity Surgery. 2016;**26**(10):2449-2456. DOI: 10.1007/s11695-016-2127-y

[51] Daher HB, Shahara AI. Gastroesophageal reflux disease, obesity, and laparoscopic sleeve gastrectomy: The burning questions. World Journal of Gastroenterology. 2019;**25**(33):4805-4813. DOI: 10.3748/wjg.v25.i33.4805

[52] Rebecchi F, Allaix ME, Patti MG, Schlottmann F, Morino M. Gastroesophageal reflux disease and morbid obesity: To sleeve or not to sleeve? World Journal of Gastroenterology. 2017;**23**(13):2269-2275. DOI: 10.3748/wjg.v23.i13.2269

[53] Evans JA, Muthusamy VR, Acosta RD, Bruining DH, Chandrasekhara V, Chathadi KV, et al. ASGE standards of practice committee. The role of endoscopy in the bariatric surgery patient. Surgery for Obesity and Related Diseases. 2015;**11**:507-517. DOI: 10.1016/j.soard.2015.02.2015

Chapter 3

The Differences between Gastroesophageal and Laryngopharyngeal Reflux

Ljiljana Širić, Marinela Rosso and Aleksandar Včev

Abstract

Gastroesophageal reflux (GER) and laryngopharyngeal reflux (LPR) have different pathophysiological mechanisms of occurrence and are characterized by different clinical pictures and symptomatology. In clinical practice, it often happens that LPR remains unrecognized or is defined as atypical gastroesophageal reflux, thus, it is necessary to distinguish between these two clinical entities. Laryngopharyngeal reflux refers to the return of gastric contents from the stomach through the esophagus to the larynx, pharynx, paranasal cavities, middle ear, and lower respiratory tract, and it is part of the wider extraesophageal reflux syndrome (EER). Extraesophageal symptoms are common in GERD, and studies show an increasing prevalence of LPR in patients with GERD, as well as an association of reflux disease with cough and dysphonia symptoms. The aim of the chapter is to describe differences between GER and LPR in order to facilitate the recognition and differentiation of manifest and latent symptoms, diagnosis, and choice of therapeutic approach.

Keywords: cough, gastroesophageal reflux, gastroesophageal reflux disease, dysphonia, dysphagia, laryngopharyngeal reflux

1. Introduction

The terms gastroesophageal reflux (GER) and laryngopharyngeal reflux (LPR) refer to the anatomical position and cause of the disease. Reflux sometimes escapes into the distal esophagus, which is a physiological event, but laryngeal mucosa does not possess protective mechanisms against gastric contents, so it appears that laryngopharyngeal reflux cannot be physiological. Gastroesophageal reflux disease (GERD) is one of the most common gastrointestinal disorders in Western countries, defined as a stomach content reflux into the esophagus with pathohistological changes of the esophageal mucous membrane and a series of clinical symptoms. The manifestations and symptoms of GERD have been classified into either esophageal or extra-esophageal. Extra-esophageal manifestations include upper respiratory tract manifestations, oral cavity, pulmonary, cardiac manifestation, and chest pain. Laryngopharyngeal reflux was conceptualized as the backflow of gastric contents into the laryngopharynx and other parts of the upper aerodigestive tract, causing an inflammatory reaction of the mucous membrane of pharynx, larynx, and other associated respiratory organs.

In recent years it has been proven that gastroesophageal reflux is not the only cause of LPR. A growing number of clinical research support the opinion of LPRD being a new clinical entity, which is different from GERD in terms of pathogenesis, clinical manifestations, diagnostic and therapeutic possibilities, and prognosis. Physicians of various professions are involved in the diagnostic and therapeutic procedures of these pathological conditions. LPR, as well as GERD, is one of the most common causes of patient visits to their family medicine physicians. For primary care physicians, those conditions represent an important medical problem and a challenge in fast diagnostics, effective treatment, and proper selection of patients who require additional multidisciplinary diagnostic procedures [1]. The development of the diseases can be benign or malignant, with a number of potential medical complications and health-threatening and life-threatening consequences, and most of its forms can greatly affect patient's quality of life.

2. Epidemiology

In recent years, the global prevalence of GERD is increasing. Based on geographical, lifestyle, and diet habits, in different regions of the world varies from 2.5% to 51.2%. According to epidemiological research, the prevalence of GERD appears to be the highest in Southeast Europe and South Asia (more than 25%), and lowest in Canada, France, and Southeast Asia (below 10%) [2]. The prevalence of laryngopharyngeal reflux has also been constantly rising in the Western world and today affects an alarmingly high percentage of the general population. It is estimated that clinical presentation of LPR could be found in 5–30% of individuals [1]. About 10% of patients visiting ENT clinics have symptoms attributed to LPR, which is present in up to 50% of patients with voice disorders [3].

Symptoms and findings are mainly nonspecific and some physicians believe that LPR is over-diagnosed. In clinical practice, the possibility of over- or under-diagnosed LPR depends on numerous factors, including physician's experience, expertise, and knowledge, as well as diagnostic methods [4].

3. Esophageal anatomy and physiology

A GER episode is diagnosed when esophageal pH drops below 4.0 for at least 30 seconds. The physiological GER occurs in normal individuals, typically postprandial. Under physiological conditions, there is a number of protective mechanisms, which prevent epithelial damage due to reflux contents. These include upper esophageal sphincter (UES), lower esophageal sphincter (LES), esophageal peristalsis, the squamous mucosal barrier, salivary production, and bicarbonate buffer. Esophageal sphincters work as physical barriers to the retrograde movement of stomach contents to the esophagus and upper airway spaces. The esophagus is a 25 cm hollow fibromuscular tube that allows the passage of solids and liquids from the pharynx to the stomach, with no metabolic, digestive or endocrine function. It makes continuation with pharynx with the upper esophageal sphincter, which measures 2–4 cm in length, and is composed of striated or skeletal muscle. The cricoid cartilage and the arytenoid and inter arytenoid muscles make up the anterior parts of the sphincter. The thyropharyngeus and the cricopharyngeus muscles form the majority of the sphincter's posterior and lateral walls, with the former accounting for the upper two-thirds of the sphincter and the latter occupying the lower one-third. Contraction of the hyoid muscle that pulls the larynx forward, linked to the relaxation of the cricopharyngeus and the thyropharyngeus, leads to sphincter opening wide.

The primary role of the UES is to protect the upper airway spaces from retrograde movement of stomach contents. It also prevents a bigger amount of air from reaching the gastrointestinal tract. Lower esophageal sphincter, which measures 2.5–3.5 cm in length, is composed of smooth muscle and is not a true anatomical sphincter, but it is a physiological sphincter that is under involuntary control by the sympathetic trunk and the vagal nerve. In response to direct inhibitory signals, the smooth muscles in the LES relax, allowing the sphincter to open, and the bolus to pass. The LES and the crural diaphragm constitute a high-pressure zone that act as a mechanical anti-reflux barrier that minimizes movement of stomach contents back into the esophagus and also allows the bolus into the stomach [5].

Esophageal peristalsis is a process of simultaneous constriction and distal relaxation, which drives the bolus toward the stomach. This process ends by relaxation and opening of the LES and enabling the passage of the bolus into the stomach. The esophagus is lined with stratified squamous epithelium. The submucosal glands secrete water, bicarbonate, mucins, epidermal growth factor, and prostaglandins. This secretion is involved in mucosal clearance. At the gastroesophageal junction is a change to simple columnar epithelial cells with gastric glands and pits. This squamocolumnar junction is of special importance in patients with reflux disease—it is a critical point for the development of Barrett's esophagus, a premalignant condition that is associated with esophageal carcinoma [6].

4. Etiopathogenesis

New diagnostic methods developed in recent decades have greatly helped to understand the pathophysiology of these conditions. Numerous studies have evaluated the multifactorial background of GERD and LPR.

4.1 Etiology and pathophysiology of GERD

Various critical factors and mechanisms are contributing to GERD: LES incompetence, hiatal hernia, and hiatal anatomic changes, protrusion or herniation of the upper part of the stomach into the thorax, an altered frequency of transient LES relaxations, esophageal acid exposure, insufficient esophageal motility, and delayed gastric emptying [7]. Diet and conditions, which increase intra-abdominal pressure such as pregnancy, obesity, and straining play a role, as well as presence of Helicobacter pylori [8]. In addition, alcohol, nicotine, caffeine, and certain medications, such as calcium channel blockers or anticholinergic agents, have been shown to cause LES incompetence, which is the main cause of GERD [9].

Many GERD patients exhibit esophageal dysmotility and prolonged clearance rates [10]. GERD and psychosocial disorders often occur together and can affect each other [11]. Obstructive sleep apnea (OSA), obstructive sleep apnea syndrome (OSAS), and GERD have a strong relationship and share several common risk factors: approximately 40–60% of patients with OSA also suffer from GERD [12].

The pathological effect of refluxed gastric contents is complex and caused by acids, pepsin, bile acids, and trypsin. The overall mechanism of cell damage is penetration of the epithelium by acids at low pH and proteolysis of collagen, which disrupts the basement membrane of the squamous epithelial cells. Acid and bile reflux play a critical role—hydrochloric acid is a major cause of esophageal irritation and reflux symptoms causing injury to mucosal epithelial cells and inflammation. The abnormal secretion and activation of pepsin can also cause proteolysis and cell damage [13]. Pathohistological changes in the esophageal mucosa can be divided into three categories: nonerosive reflux disease, reflux oesophagitis, and Barett's esophagus [14].

4.2 Etiology and pathophysiology of LPRD

The pathophysiology of LPR is still incompletely understood. In the contrast to GERD, as we have already noted, LPR is never physiological, and mucosa of the upper respiratory tract is not resistant to gastric content. Although dysfunction of any previously mentioned barrier can cause LPR, the pathophysiology of LPR is primarily attributed to failure or dysfunction of the upper esophageal sphincter. The retrograde flow of gastric acid and pepsin induces mucosal inflammatory reaction and overall cell damage. Tripsin makes role in LES abnormalities and heat sensitivity disturbing barrier function. Furthermore, stress and autonomic nerve dysfunction by increasing the opening of LES and UES are probably involved in the development of LPR. In some studies, it has been hypothesized that gas refluxes carry aerosolized droplets containing hydrogen and pepsin into the proximal esophagus and upper respiratory space. Microaspiration of acid droplets is a very important mechanism for the development of mucosal inflammation [15].

4.3 Pathophysiological differences

Esophageal mucosa is more resistant to acid attacks, a critical pH is 4.0, cell death and mucosal injury occur below this point. Laryngeal mucosa damage occurs at a pH of 5.0 with short-term exposure. Laryngeal epithelium is up to 100 times more sensitive to pepsin damage than esophageal tissues, and according to some authors, it seems that pepsin plays a key role in the pathogenesis of laryngopharyngeal reflux [16]. Up to 50 GER episodes per day are considered within the normal range; however, LPR more than 3 times a week can lead to pathological changes in the laryngopharyngeal region [17]. GERD is associated with a higher body mass index (BMI), which is not observed in LPR [18]. As can be observed, GERD and LPR have some different etiological and pathogenic features, as shown in **Table 1**.

	GERD	**LPR**
Etiology	LES	UES
Critical pH	4.0	5.0
Esophageal motility	impaired	normal
Reflux	liquid	gas
Obesity	yes	no
Critical number of reflux episodes	>50/day	>3/week

Table 1.
Comparison of GERD and LPR based on etiology and pathogenesis.

	GERD	LPR
Heartburn	Yes	Uncommon
Acid reflux	Yes	Uncommon
Position	Supine	Upright
Occurrence	Anytime	Daytime
Sleep Disorders	OSAS	Insomnia

Table 2.
Comparison of GERD and LPR based on main symptoms.

5. Symptoms

GERD patients usually present with wide symptoms of esophagitis, including heartburn and burning sensation, chest pain, and acid regurgitation, which are important diagnostic factors. Patients mainly report a burning feeling in the retrosternal area, spreading into the chest and neck. It occurs mostly post-prandially. Chronic cough, dysphagia, globus sensation, and irritable throat discomfort can present as atypical manifestations in patients with GERD as extraesophageal symptoms. Some patients with GERD are asymptomatic. Some clinical studies show that reflux is the only cause of chronic cough in 10% of patients [19].

The most prevalent symptoms associated with LPR are related to the upper respiratory tract: globus sensation, hoarseness, throat clearing, excess throat mucus or postnasal drip. These symptoms, which are commonly observed in primary care medicine, are nonspecific and often intermittent. Throat pain, sore throat, expectoration, dysphagia, and halitosis can also be presented [1]. Patients with LPR are more likely to suffer from insomnia [20].

GERD symptoms typically occur in supine position, but LPR patients mainly have upright and daytime reflux events [21]. The main differences in clinical presentation are shown in **Table 2**.

6. Diagnosis

A presumptive diagnosis of GERD is based on typical symptomatology. Empirical proton-pump inhibitor (PPI) treatment, where the patient is prescribed a PPI for a short period of time (usually two months) to see if it resolves symptoms is in the majority of patients sufficient for diagnosis of GERD. In case when symptoms do not improve, or even worsen, when GERD is accompanied with other, atypical symptoms or, in case of suspected complications, there is a need for more invasive diagnostic tests.

While routine endoscope examination of the esophagus is not indicated for patients with typical symptoms, it is advised for patients with complicated GERD and is useful in the detection of erosive esophagitis, presence of Barett's esophagus or hiatal hernia, and other anatomic changes. The absence of esophageal mucosal injury cannot exclude GERD, because more than half of the patients with GERD have nonerosive reflux disease [22]. Routine biopsy is not recommended. The detection rate of abnormal blood vessels and epithelial micro injuries can be improved under endoscopy equipped with narrow banding imaging [22]. Barium esophagography and pH monitoring are useful to evaluate esophageal function. Esophageal manometry is of limited value but is recommended before considering anti-reflux surgery. Ambulatory reflux monitoring allows the determination of pathologic esophageal acid reflux and its frequency [23]. Blood tests are used to measure H. pylori IgG and H. pylori CagA IgG antibodies.

Standard diagnostic algorithm, which could precisely determine LPR have still not been established. LPR is mostly not recognized, and because of that it is known as a "silent reflux." In a large number of cases diagnostic and therapeutical protocols are inadequate, so proper treatment is usually delayed. Laryngeal symptoms are most common, so patients are usually treated by otolaryngologists. Otolaryngologists have developed a Reflux Symptom Index (RSI), a validated questionnaire given to patients to score the severity of their symptoms. It is based on the importance of certain disease symptoms (the degree of hoarseness, frequency of throat clearing, degree of throat mucus or postnasal drip, dysphagia, coughing after eating or lying down, breathing difficulties, chronic cough, globus sensation, and heartburn). Reflux Finding Score (RFS) is based on frequency of pathological changes observed by laryngoscopy [24]. The laryngoscopic findings associated with LPR include posterior commissure hypertrophy, edema, arytenoid erythema, ventricular obliteration, granulation, oropharyngeal and anterior pilar erythema, coated tongue, uvula, and oropharyngeal posterior wall erythema. Many of them are nonspecific, but laryngoscopy has a very important role in diagnosis of reflux laryngitis; redness, thickness, and swelling located in the posterior parts of the larynx (posterior laryngitis) are important for the diagnosis of LPR.

This part of the larynx is anatomically more disposed to chronic irritation because both arytenoids and the interarytenoid regions are closer to the inlet of esophagus [25]. In some cases, immunoserologic pepsin detection tests are useful and easy to perform. Pepsin is produced only by the chief cells of the stomach and, therefore, the pepsin as a specific marker detected in the larynx can only be derived from refluxing gastric contents [26].

7. Differential diagnosis

GERD symptoms overlap with those of other pathological conditions:

- Infectious esophagitis;
- Eosinophilic esophagitis;
- Peptic ulcer disease;
- Gastroparesis;
- Esophageal motor disorders;
- Esophageal stricture;
- Esophageal cancer;
- Coronary artery disease;
- Biliary colic;

- Functional dyspepsia;
- Dysphagia;
- Various pulmonary diseases [23].

Many diseases and conditions of the upper respiratory tract can be presented as LPR and can be easily attributed to them:

- Postnasal drip;
- Allergies;
- Chronic laryngitis;
- Sinus inflammation;
- Vocal fold pathology;
- Various pulmonary diseases;
- Zenker's diverticulum;
- Laryngeal and pharyngeal malignancies [27].

This poses a challenge to diagnosis and can alter medical treatment.

8. Treatment

Dietary changes and lifestyle modifications are the first steps in the treatment of GERD. This includes eating low-fat and low-acid diet, small meal size, weight loss, smoking cessation, and controlling alcohol consumption. Stress management is also useful. Patients with nocturnal reflux have to eat a meal 2–3 h before bedtime and elevate the head of the bed during sleep. If these measures fail to achieve results, the widely accepted empirical management of LFR and GERD is proton pump inhibitor (PPI) treatment applied twice a day for two or three months. These drugs can suppress acid production and neutralize acidopeptidic activity in esophagus, larynx, and pharynx. PPIs are fast and strong, and the most efficacious and important factor for success of the therapy is their regular and correct usage. Patients who need PPI therapy for a longer time should be placed on the lowest dose because the long-term use of PPIs increases the risk of many complications, such as acute nephritis, gastric tumors, bacterial gastroenteritis, bone fractures, etc. [23, 28].

H2 receptor blockers are an effective alternative maintenance therapy for GERD and LPR, as well as alginates. Alginate forms a gelatinous layer on top of the gastric contents and makes a mechanical barrier, thereby reducing contact between the reflux contents and esophageal mucosa. Alginate also has a significant inhibitory effect on pepsin, and is, according to some research, non-inferior to PPI [13, 29]. Other noninvasive treatment options include using external upper esophageal sphincter compression device. If there is no response to appropriate empirical treatment, instead of increasing the dose or extending the duration of treatment, it is necessary to review the diagnosis by considering the multifactorial pathophysiology of reflux. In patients with severe reflux, surgical therapy can also be used. Endoscopic and surgical options include anti-reflux surgery, bariatric surgery, magnetic sphincter augmentation, and transoral incisionless fundoplication [22]. As can be seen, the medicament treatment of GERD and LPR is similar, but in clinical practice, patients with LPR require more aggressive and prolonged PPI treatments (six months) to achieve an improvement of laryngeal symptoms than those with typical GERD symptoms [30].

9. Complications

As already stated, untreated or unrecognized reflux episodes can be connected with a number of potential medical complications and health-threatening and life-threatening consequences. The prevalent complications of GERD include dysphagia, bleeding from erosive esophagitis, and esophageal adenocarcinoma. Dysphagia usually occurs slowly in patients with long-standing heartburn. The most common causes are peptic stricture and severe inflammation, but dysphagia can be the first symptom of pathological esophageal mucosa changes and esophageal cancer. It is considered an alarming symptom in patients with GERD that requires endoscopy [31].

Severe esophagitis is a risk factor for development of Barett's esophagus (BE). Barrett's esophagus is a condition defined as a metaplastic transformation of the distal normal esophageal squamous epithelium into the columnar epithelium. It is considered a premalignant condition, the only known predisposing factor of epithelial dysplasia and esophageal carcinoma. Long-term and non-treated gastroesophageal reflux disease is the most important risk factor for the development of this condition. BE is found in 1.3–1.6% of the general population and 5–15% of symptomatic GERD patients undergoing endoscopy.

The incidence of GERD has been increasing significantly over the last few decades, as well as incidence of adenocarcinoma of the esophagus. As BE is the only known precursor to carcinoma, progress in the monitoring and therapy of BE are essential to enable early diagnosis and improve patient outcomes.

Lower esophageal rings (Schatzki) correlate with reflux esophagitis, too. Other complications include anemia (due to chronic blood loss), peptic ulceration, and a whole range of respiratory tract problems [32].

Laryngeal and pharyngeal mucosa has a poor self-protection capacity and poor adaptability to chemical stimuli. Some significant long-term complications of LPR are chronic otitis media, chronic rhinosinusitis, oral cavity disorders and dental erosions, recurrent bronchopulmonary infections, and cardiac problems. More serious, but not so often, laryngeal findings in patients with LPR include vocal cord nodules, laryngospasms, subglottic stenosis, and arytenoid fixation. LPR is also an independent risk factor for squamous cancer of the larynx and pharynx. Pepsin has been linked to epithelial proliferation and carcinogenesis. Namely, activated pepsin induces inflammation, destruction of the epithelial defense barrier, changes in expression of laryngeal and hypopharyngeal genes and tumorogenesis, and disruption of the function of epithelial cells [33–36]. Some studies have shown that bile acids and Helicobacter pylori may play a role in the development of laryngeal and hypopharyngeal carcinoma.

10. Prognosis

Majority of patients with GERD and LPR do well with medications, but relapse after stopping medical treatment is common. In refractory cases, surgical treatment is necessary. Long-term untreated LPR, as well as GERD, can result in previously mentioned complications.

11. Conclusion

Different results of scientific studies make it difficult to establish clear approach to the symptoms and manifestations of LPR and its relation to GERD. The multifactorial pathophysiology of reflux needs to be investigated in more detail [37]. GERD typically manifests as heartburn, regurgitation, and chest pain, while LPR patients usually do not report these symptoms, and they complain about chronic cough, laryngitis, and a lump in the throat. According to some investigations, ≤50% of LPR patients have GERD, while laryngopharyngeal symptoms were present in 32.8% of GERD patients. LPR patients mainly have gaseous, upright, and daytime reflux events, and only 5.5% of laryngopharyngeal reflux events occurred at nighttime, in the supine position.

GERD could be diagnosed using multiple tools, but fewer objective diagnostic tools exist for diagnosing LPR. However, up to 50% of patients with LPR symptoms may not have classic reflux symptoms. The interindividual differences in the esophageal and laryngopharyngeal mucosa sensitivity must be taken into account, too. The esophagoscopy may be normal in more than 44% of cases and may detect esophagitis in 10–30% of LPR patients, while erosive esophagitis is found in almost 50% of GERD patients. Scientific evidence shows that LPR is not an advanced stage of GERD [17].

The independent existence of LPR in the absence of GERD can be understood through several possibilities. First, reflux can originate from the heterotopic gastric mucosa of the cervical esophagus. Second, reflux events detected in the laryngopharynx are secondary to GER, and patients met both of diagnostic criteria. Third, reflux events detected only in the laryngopharynx are secondary to GER and meet the diagnostic criteria for LPR, but do not meet the criteria for GERD. It seems that more studies would make it possible to define the reflux standard for GERD as well as put together the standard differentiation between LPR and GERD [38].

Safe standard diagnostic procedures, which could precisely determine LPR, have still not been established, and taking careful and detailed hetero-anamnestic history is important. In GERD, typical reflux symptoms usually regress with antireflux therapy, but several meta-analyses have demonstrated no diagnostic or therapeutic benefit of PPI to manage patients with LPRD. Therefore, establishing a multidisciplinary collaboration between gastroenterologists, laryngologists, family medicine physicians, pediatricians, pulmonologists, psychiatrists, and speech-language pathologists is necessary to provide a comprehensive approach to develop acceptable diagnostic and treatment modalities for the pathologic reflux.

A generally accepted view today is that, although the relationship between them is not completely understood, it is necessary to consider them as different types of medical entities and treat them in a different way. Anyway, GERD and LPR can coexist with each other and also independently as different subheadings under the main heading reflux disease [17].

Conflict of interest

The authors declare no conflict of interest.

Author details

Ljiljana Širić[1,2]*, Marinela Rosso[3] and Aleksandar Včev[4,5]

1 Department of Otorhinolaryngology and Head and Neck Surgery, University Hospital Center Osijek, Osijek, Croatia

2 Faculty of Kinesiology, Department of General and Applied Kinesiology, University of Zagreb, Zagreb, Croatia

3 Polyclinic Rosso, Osijek, Croatia

4 Faculty of Dental Medicine and Health, J.J. Strossmayer University of Osijek, Osijek, Croatia

5 Faculty of Medicine, Department of Pathophysiology, J.J. Strossmayer University of Osijek, Osijek, Croatia

*Address all correspondence to: ljsiric@gmail.com

References

[1] Lechien JR, Saussez S, Muls V, Barillari MR, Chiesa-Estomba CM, Hans S, et al. Laryngopharyngeal reflux: A state-of-the-art algorithm management for primary care physicians. Journal of Clinical Medicine. 2020;**9**(11):3618

[2] Richter JE, Rubenstein JH. Presentation and epidemiology of gastroesophageal reflux disease. Gastroenterology. 2018;**154**(2):267-276

[3] Koufman JA. The otolaryngologic manifestations of gastroesophageal reflux disease (GERD): A clinical investigation of 225 patients using ambulatory 24-hour pH monitoring and an experimental investigation of the role of acid and pepsin in the development of laryngeal injury. Laryngoscope. 1991;**101**:1-78

[4] Chang BA, MacNeil SD, Morrison MD, Lee PK. The reliability of the reflux finding score among general otolaryngologists. Journal of Voice. 2015;**29**:572-577

[5] Bajwa SA, Toro F, Kasi A. Physiology, Esophagus. Treasure Island: StatPearls; 2022

[6] Naini BV, Chak A, Ali MA, Odze RD. Barrett's oesophagus diagnostic criteria: Endoscopy and histology. Best Practice & Research. Clinical Gastroenterology. 2015;**29**(1):77-96

[7] Fuchs KH, Lee AM, Breithaupt W, Varga G, Babic B, Horgan S. Pathophysiology of gastroesophageal reflux disease-which factors are important? Translational Gastroenterology and Hepatology. 2021;**6**:53

[8] Wang FW, Tu MS, Chuang HY, Yu HC, Cheng LC, Hsu PI. Erosive esophagitis in asymptomatic subjects: Risk factors. Digestive Diseases and Sciences. 2010;**55**(5):1320-1324

[9] Allen M, Mellow M, Robinson MG, Orr WC. Comparison of calcium channel blocking agents and an anticholinergic agent on oesophageal function. Alimentary Pharmacology & Therapeutics. 1987;**1**(2):153-159

[10] Postma G, Tomek M, Belafsky P, Kaufman J. Esophageal motor function in laryngopharyngeal reflux is superior to that in classic gastroesophageal reflux disease. The Annals of Otology, Rhinolology, and Laryngology. 2011;**110**(12):1114-1116

[11] He M, Wang Q, Yao D, Li J, Bai G. Association between psychosocial disorders and gastroesophageal reflux disease: A systematic review and meta-analysis. Journal of Neurogastroenterology and Motility. 2022;**28**(2):212-221

[12] Mahfouz R, Barchuk A, Obeidat AE, Mansour MM, Hernandez D, Darweesh M, et al. The relationship between obstructive sleep apnea (OSA) and gastroesophageal reflux disease (GERD) in inpatient settings: A Nationwide Study. Cureus. 2022;**14**(3):e22810

[13] Li Y, Xu G, Zhou B, Tang Y, Liu X, Wu Y, et al. Effects of acids, pepsin, bile acids, and trypsin on laryngopharyngeal reflux diseases: Physiopathology and therapeutic targets. European Archives of Oto-Rhino-Laryngology. 2022;**279**(6):2743-2752

[14] Zhang D, Liu S, Li Z, Wang R. Global, regional and national burden of gastroesophageal reflux disease,

1990-2019: Update from the GBD 2019 study. Annals of Medicine. 2022;**54**(1):1372-1384

[15] de Bortoli N, Nacci A, Savarino E, Martinucci I, Bellini M, Fattori B, et al. How many cases of laryngopharyngeal reflux suspected by laryngoscopy are gastroesophageal reflux disease-related? World Journal of Gastroenterology. 2012;**18**(32):4363-4370

[16] Samuels TL, Johnston N. Pepsin as a causal agent of inflammation during nonacidic reflux. Otolaryngology and Head and Neck Surgery. 2009;**141**(5):559-563

[17] Sirin S, Öz F. Laryngopharyngeal reflux concept: What is known and what should we focus on? Brazilian Journal of Otorhinolaryngology. 2019;**85**(2):133-135

[18] Vincent DA Jr, Garrett JD, Radionoff SL, Reussner LA, Stasney CR. The proximal probe in esophageal pH monitoring: Development of a normative database. Journal of Voice. 2000;**14**(2):247-254

[19] Benini L, Ferrari M, Sembenini C, Olivieri M, Micciolo R, Zuccali V, et al. Cough threshold in reflux oesophagitis: Influence of acid and of laryngeal and oesophageal damage. Gut. 2000;**46**(6):762-767

[20] Kang JW, Park JM, Lee YC, Eun YG. The association between laryngopharyngeal reflux and insomnia. European Archives of Oto-Rhino-Laryngology. 2022;**279**(7):3535-3541

[21] Belafsky PC, Postma GN, Koufman JA. Laryngopharyngeal reflux symptoms improve before changes in physical findings. The Laryngoscope. 2001;**111**(6):979-981

[22] Chen S, Du F, Zhong C, Liu C, Wang X, Chen Y, et al. Gastroesophageal reflux disease: Recent innovations in endoscopic assessment and treatment. Gastroenterology Report (Oxf). 2021;**9**(5):383-391

[23] Azer SA, Reddivari AKR. Reflux Esophagitis. Treasure Island (FL): StatPearls; 2022

[24] Junaid M, Qadeer Ahmed S, Kazi M, Khan HU, Sohail HM. Laryngopharyngeal reflux disease: Outcome of patients after treatment in otolaryngology clinics. Cureus. 2020;**12**(12):e12195

[25] Du C, Thayer P, Yan Y, Liu Q, Wang L, Jiang J. Changing trends of color of different laryngeal regions in laryngopharyngeal reflux disease. Ear, Nose, & Throat Journal. 2020;**99**(8):543-547

[26] Guo Z, Jiang J, Wu H, Zhu J, Zhang S, Zhang C. Salivary peptest for laryngopharyngeal reflux and gastroesophageal reflux disease: A systemic review and meta-analysis. Medicine (Baltimore). 2021;**100**(32):e26756

[27] Barry DW, Vaezi MF. Laryngopharyngeal reflux: More questions than answers. Cleveland Clinic Journal of Medicine. 2010;**77**(5):327-334

[28] Kahrilas PJ, Shaheen NJ, Vaezi MF. American Gastroenterological Association Institute; Clinical Practice and Quality Management Committee. American Gastroenterological Association Institute technical review on the management of gastroesophageal reflux disease. Gastroenterology. 2008;**135**(4):1392-1413

[29] Pizzorni N, Ambrogi F, Eplite A, Rama S, Robotti C, Lechien J, et al. Magnesium alginate versus proton pump inhibitors for the treatment of laryngopharyngeal reflux: A

non-inferiority randomized controlled trial. European Archives of Oto-Rhino-Laryngology. 2022;**279**(5):2533-2542

[30] Salihefendic N, Zildzic M, Cabric E. Laryngopharyngeal reflux disease - LPRD. Medieval Archaeology. 2017;**71**(3):215-218

[31] Khieu M, Mukherjee S. Barrett Esophagus. Treasure Island: StatPearls; 2022

[32] Brown J, Shermetaro C. Laryngopharyngeal Reflux. Treasure Island, FL: StatPearls; 2022

[33] Ward PH, Hanson DG. Reflux as an etiological factor of carcinoma of the laryngopharynx. The Laryngoscope. 1988;**98**(11):1195-1199

[34] Širić Lj, Rosso M, Včev A. Extraesophageal manifestations and symptoms of esophageal diseases. In: Neri V, Ahmed M. editors. Esophagitis and Gastritis—Recent Updates. London: IntechOpen; 2021

[35] Yin CY, Zhang SS, Zhong JT, Zhou SH. Pepsin and laryngeal and hypopharyngeal carcinomas. Clinical Experiment in Otorhinolaryngology. 2021;**14**(2):159-168

[36] Huang Y, Gu M, Wu Q, Zhu J, Wu J, Wang P, et al. Is laryngeal squamous cell carcinoma related to Helicobacter pylori? Frontiers in Oncology. 2022;**12**:790997

[37] Külekçi S, Ertugay ÇK, Toros SZ. The effects of empiric antireflux treatment on laryngopharyngeal and gastroesophageal reflux disease. Sisli Etfal Hastanesi Tip Bulteni. 2020;**54**(1):29-35

[38] Wu Y, Wang J, Huang Q, Peng T, Zhao L, Feng G, et al. The relationship between gastroesophageal reflux disease and laryngopharyngeal reflux based on pH monitoring. Ear, Nose, & Throat Journal. 2021;**100**(4):249-253

Chapter 4

Review of Gastroesophageal Reflux Pharmacotherapy Management

Anthony Wilks, Ladan Panahi, George Udeani and Salim Surani

Abstract

Acid suppressive therapy (AST) has been the primary mechanism to provide gastroesophageal reflux disease (GERD) symptomatic relief and prevent complications in many individuals with GERD. Many AST options exist, but proton pump inhibitors (PPIs) have developed popularity in symptomatic relief for refractory GERD patients. To help reduce persistent symptoms, the use of AST therapy optimization is imperative and involves timing doses appropriately and increasing the dose and dosing frequency. Recently, more data has become available regarding the safety profile of AST, specifically PPI use. This data has raised awareness about its potential for toxicity with long-term use. This chapter focuses on the pharmacological management of GERD with a focus on the current updates regarding AST safety and efficacy.

Keywords: histamine 2 receptor antagonists, proton pump inhibitors, acid suppressive therapy, antacids, GERD, gastroesophageal reflux disease

1. Introduction

Gastroesophageal reflux disorder (GERD) is one of the most prevalent digestive disorders in the United States and affects almost 28% of the American population [1, 2]. GERD is a chronic condition that occurs when acid flows from the stomach back up into the esophagus, which causes the upper digestive tract mucosal lining to become irritated [3]. There are many common causes of GERD, including alcohol, obesity, spicy foods, medications, hiatal hernias, and pregnancy [4]. Heartburn, one of the most common symptoms of GERD, is a form of indigestion that typically produces a burning sensation in the chest region due to acid reflux [2]. Other less common symptoms of GERD include frequent burping, pain upon swallowing, a sore or hoarse throat, cough, a sensation of a lump in the throat, and asthma. GERD can lead to serious long-term complications such as Barrett's esophagus, erosive esophagitis, or esophageal cancer if left untreated, which makes treating the condition important [5]. Once patients have an established clinical diagnosis of GERD, treatment options include medications, lifestyle modifications, and surgery. Therapy goals include eliminating symptoms, managing and preventing complications, and maintaining remission [6]. Lifestyle modifications are an essential treatment component, including dietary changes such as decreasing consumption of fatty and spicy foods and reducing caffeine intake. Others include exercising, reducing weight, avoiding smoking, and head elevation while resting or sleeping [7]. Acid-suppressive therapy (AST), such as proton pump inhibitors (PPIs), histamine two receptor antagonists (H2RA), and antacids, are the cornerstone of treatment for GERD. Since GERD is a chronic disease, lifelong treatment is typically necessary to reduce symptoms and prevent long-term complications [8].

2. Antacid therapy

Antacids are medications that neutralize stomach acid, thereby increasing gastric pH [9]. Common brands of antacids, which are available over-the-counter, include Maalox®, Rolaids®, Tums®, and Gaviscon® [9]. The various properties of these different products are listed in **Table 1** [9]. Antacids are available in different formulations, which commonly include aluminum, calcium, or magnesium salts. Aluminum hydroxide and magnesium hydroxide salts neutralize gastric acid, forming aluminum or magnesium salts and water. The antacids increase gastric pH and inhibit pepsin activity [9]. Aluminum hydroxide's therapeutic effect is 20–60 minutes when fasting or up to 3 hours, taking effect 1 hour after meals [9]. Magnesium hydroxide's duration of action occurs from 30 minutes to 6 hours after administration [9]. Calcium salts

Medication	Formulation	Dosage	Duration
Calcium carbonate	Tablet 1 g	1–4 tablets by mouth with a maximum of 8 g/day as calcium carbonate as symptoms occur.	14 days
Calcium carbonate and magnesium hydroxide	Chewable tablets: 700 mg/300 mg	Chew 2–4 tablets by mouth four times a day with a maximum of 8 tablets per 24 hours	14 days
Calcium carbonate and magnesium hydroxide	Liquid: 400 mg/135 mg per 5 ml	Take 10–20 ml by mouth four times a day with a maximum of 90 ml per 24 hours	14 days
Aluminum hydroxide, magnesium hydroxide, and simethicone	Tablets: 200 mg/200 mg/25 mg Liquid: 200 mg/200 mg/20 mg per 5 ml Liquid:400 mg/400 mg/200 mg per 5 ml	Take 1–4 tablets four times a day as needed with a maximum of 16 tablets in 24 hours Take 10–20 ml between each meal and at bedtime, or as directed by your physician, with a maximum of 120 ml per 24 hours	14 days
Aluminum hydroxide and magnesium trisilicate	Chewable tablet: 80 mg/14.2 mg	Chew 2–4 tablets four times a day with a maximum of 16 tablets per 24 hours	14 days

Table 1.
Dosing and duration of available antacids [5, 6, 10, 11].

work by inhibiting the proteolytic activity of pepsin and additionally increase the tone of the lower esophageal sphincter (LES) when pH is >4 [9]. Calcium carbonate absorbs primarily in the duodenum and changes with age (60% for infants, 28% for prepubertal children, 34% for pubertal children, and 25% for adults). It is important to note that absorption doubles during pregnancy [9]. Solubility of calcium carbonate increases with increasing acidity [9]. Constipation, diarrhea, nausea, vomiting, and hypophosphatemia are common side effects of antacid use [9]. Drug interactions with antacids are common and may involve interactions with medications such as levothyroxine, fluoroquinolones, tetracyclines, iron supplements, and salicylates. These interactions typically result in decreased absorption of the aforementioned medications and can affect therapy [9]. In order to minimize the effects of antacids on the absorption of other medications, the recommendation is to administer the medications 2 hours before or up to 6 hours after taking antacids [9]. Historically, antacids were the first-line medication for the treatment of peptic ulcer disease (PUD) prior to the introduction of PPIs [9]. Due to their familiarity and low cost, antacids are still very commonly used to treat heartburn. When used for the treatment of heartburn, patients are recommended to consult their physician if symptoms persist after 14 days of use. Antacids represent a low-cost, relatively safe option for patients with intermittent GERD symptoms but have the potential to mask more serious problems, which is why long-term unsupervised use is not recommended [9].

The use of antacids in renal dysfunction can lead to the accumulation of aluminum and magnesium. Accumulation begins when creatinine clearance (CrCl) is less than 25 ml/min, and use is not recommended when CrCl < 10 ml/min. No current dose adjustments are recommended to prevent accumulation for those with renal dysfunction [10]. For patients on hemodialysis, antacids should not be used unless patients can be reliably monitored, including signs and symptoms of toxicity and serum magnesium levels. Symptoms of hypermagnesemia include anorexia and nausea due to magnesium's depressant effect on the central nervous system.

Additionally, hypermagnesemia can cause to skeletal muscle weakness and decreased deep tendon reflexes [11, 12]. Other signs of magnesium toxicity include electrocardiographic changes, muscle weakness, and hypotension [11, 12]. Aluminum accumulation can lead to 'dialysis dementia' (impaired cognition), dialysis osteomalacia, and dialysis encephalopathy [11, 12].

3. Histamine 2 receptor antagonists (H2RA)

H2RAs consist of famotidine, ranitidine, cimetidine, and nizatidine [13]. Famotidine and cimetidine, available over the counter, are the only H2RAs currently available in the United States. The dosing and duration of these H2RAs are summarized in **Table 2** [13].

Ranitidine and nizatidine are no longer available in the United States. They were withdrawn from the market in April 2020 due to the detection of a carcinogenic agent N-nitrosodimethylamine (NDMA), in some available products [13]. NDMA is a probable human carcinogen and has been linked to multiple cancers, including kidney cancer, bladder cancer, and cancers of the digestive tract [14]. Higher concentrations of NDMA were found in older products and products stored above room temperature [14].

As food enters the stomach, the hormone gastrin is released, leading to histamine's release. Histamine binds to H2 receptors on parietal cells, activating adenylate cyclase

Drug	Formulation	Dosage	Duration
Famotidine	PO or IV	20–40 mg BID 20 mg Q12H	14 days
Cimetidine	PO or IV	400 mg QID 800 BID 300 mg Q6H	14 days

Table 2.
Dosing and duration of available H2RA.

to increase cAMP within the cell [15]. Increase in intracellular cAMP leads to protein kinase A (PKA) activation, which phosphorylates proteins, leading to the H+/K+ ATPase releasing acid into the stomach [15]. H2RAs function by competitively inhibiting H2 receptors located on the outer surface of parietal cells in the stomach's inner lining [15, 16]. By blocking the H2 receptor, H2RAs prevent the downstream effect of the release of gastric acid into the stomach [15]. This mechanism of action leads to a decrease in stomach acidity, which helps relieve the symptoms of GERD. The H2RAs are considered interchangeable as all have shown equivalent efficacy at approved doses in clinical trials [15].

All H2RAs are available as oral tablets [15]. Famotidine comes in other formulations, including a chewable tablet, a powder for oral suspension, and a solution for intravenous administration [15]. Famotidine is also available in combination with calcium carbonate, magnesium hydroxide, and ibuprofen [15]. H2RA's therapeutic effect typically begins one hour after administration, and its effect can last between 4 and 10 hours [15].

H2RAs are metabolized in the liver and the kidneys, and dose adjustments are required for renal impairment [15]. Cimetidine dose adjustments are necessary for patients with a CrCl of less than 30 ml/min. For famotidine, a dose adjustment should be made for patients with a CrCl less than 50 ml/min, as QTc prolongation has been reported in patients with renal dysfunction [15].

H2RAs have a strong safety profile due to their wide therapeutic index [15]. Reported side effects of H2RAs include constipation, diarrhea, headache, dry mouth, and abdominal pain [15]. In patients over 50 and those with renal or hepatic dysfunction, central nervous system (CNS) side effects have been observed [15]. These include anxiety, depression, confusion, insomnia, disorientation, delirium, hallucinations, and agitation [17]. Compared to famotidine, cimetidine has shown to have more side effects which are attributed to its prolonged half-life. Additionally, it has been found to have weak anti-androgenic activity. Consequently, endocrine dysfunction has been reported with cimetidine use and includes symptoms such as decreased libido, gynecomastia, impotence, hyperprolactinemia, and galactorrhea [18]. These adverse effects are more likely to occur with high-dose therapy used in hypersecretory conditions and typically do not begin to appear until at least one month of treatment [18].

For patients in the hospital setting, those who are taking H2RAs and also recceing antibiotic therapy have been found to have an elevated risk for *Clostridioides difficile* infection [19]. Additionally, increasing evidence suggests a link between AST and community- and hospital-acquired pneumonia [20]. There have been several proposed mechanisms for this association [20]. A potential mechanism for this observation is that the stomach's acidic environment, which typically serves as a barrier against pathogens, is no longer effective due to the increased pH from AST. This higher pH makes the stomach more hospitable for the pathogenic organisms to grow [20]. Additionally, some have proposed that since gastric acid usually may stimulate the cough reflex, allowing for the clearing of infectious agents from the respiratory tract, an increase in pH leads to a decrease in this mechanism of clearing pathogens [20]. Finally, another proposed mechanism is AST causing a decreased immune response due to the potential impairment of white blood cells [20].

As with other medications, there are several drug interactions with H2RAs [15]. Since H2RAs increase gastric pH, they may affect medications that require an acidic environment for proper absorption [15]. Some medications requiring an acidic environment for absorption include itraconazole, ketoconazole, ampicillin, cephalosporins, sulfonylureas, dasatinib, iron salts, gefitinib, enteric-coated budesonide, and cyanocobalamin. Additionally, cimetidine inhibits several CYP450 isoenzymes (CYP1A2, CYP3A4, CYP2C19, and CYP2D6) and thus should be avoided while taking other medications metabolized by these enzymes [15]. Examples of such drugs include warfarin, selective serotonin reuptake inhibitors (SSRIs), and theophylline [15]. Consequently, famotidine has become the preferred H2RA for GERD due to lesser side effects and lesser drug interactions compared with cimetidine [15].

While PPIs are preferred over H2RAs due to more robust evidence for their use, H2RAs can be added to PPI monotherapy in certain situations [4, 16, 21]. If there is objective evidence of night-time reflux, H2RA therapy can be added at bedtime to PPI monotherapy taken during the day in select patients. However, tachyphylaxis may develop after several weeks of use [4]. Since basal acid secretion is highest in the evening, H2RA administration in the evening may be beneficial. Additionally, H2RAs may also play a role in PPI step-down therapy. Finally, tachyphylaxis is a concern for H2Ras, if administered consecutively for 14 days or more and has also been linked to extended H2RA treatment [4].

4. Proton pump inhibitors (PPIs)

PPIs, currently available on the market, include omeprazole (Prilosec®), esomeprazole (Nexium®), lansoprazole (Prevacid®), dexlansoprazole (Dexilant®), pantoprazole (Protonix®), and rabeprazole (Aciphex®). PPIs are available both over-the-counter or via a prescription and are widely used to manage GERD, treatment/prevention of PUD, dyspepsia, pyrosis, *H. pylori* eradication, NSAID-induced ulcers, and erosive esophagitis [22].

PPIs irreversibly bind to the (H+, K+)-ATPase enzyme in the stomach's parietal cells, preventing gastric acid (H+) release [23]. PPIs are prodrugs converted to the active form (sulphenamide) of the drug via protonation by hydrogen ions in the gastric acid [24]. Dexlansoprazole (Dexilant®), the R-enantiomer of lansoprazole, is available as a unique dual delayed-release formulation. Dexlansoprazole is currently the only dual delayed-release formulation of a PPI commercially available in the United States [25]. Dexlansoprazole capsules contain two sets of enteric-coated granules designed to disintegrate at different pH levels [25]. The first set of granules begins to disintegrate in the proximal small intestine and the second set disintegrates at a higher pH further down the intestinal tract [25].

PPIs are the recommended first-line agents for pharmacological management of GERD. An 8-week course of therapy is recommended to provide symptomatic relief and allows healing of erosive esophagitis [4]. All PPIs are considered clinically equivalent; therefore, any agent is acceptable as a first-line option [4]. Once a day, dosing before the first meal of the day is recommended initially for most PPIs [25]. Administering traditional delayed-release PPIs 30–60 minutes prior to meals is preferred in order to obtain optimal pH control. Administration of PPIs before meals allow the prodrug to be converted to the active sulphenamide form via gastric acid [26]. In contrast, newer formulations such as Dexilant® do not have to be administered regarding meals, allowing for dosing flexibility [4]. If a patient only has a partial response to PPI therapy, it is recommended to either change the timing of the dose or switch to a different PPI [4]. If neither of these changes is effective, further options include increasing the PPI from once to twice daily, primarily if the patient reports night-time symptoms or sleep disturbances [4]. Alternatively, a trial of dexlansoprazole can be considered due to its unique release mechanism, which may help reduce breakthrough symptoms [25]. Maintenance therapy beyond the initial 8 weeks can be considered if the patient continues to be symptomatic after completion of therapy or has complications such as Barrett's esophagus or erosive esophagitis [4]. The lowest effective dose possible should always be used to avoid complications and long-term side effects [4].

Typical side-effects include headache, diarrhea, nausea, vomiting, and abdominal pain. PPIs' potentially more severe side effects include hypomagnesemia, B12 deficiency, increased risk of osteoporosis-related fractures, and *C. difficile* infections. PPIs should not be used long-term unless instructed by the patient's provider to minimize the risk of the severe side effects mentioned above. Other potential risks include reduced nutrient absorption, dementia, and an increased risk of pneumonia [27].

The reduction of gastric acid due to PPI use may result in decreased absorption of vitamin B12 (cyanocobalamin), iron, and calcium salts [28]. It is recommended for patients to be monitored for pernicious anemia while on PPI therapy [28].

As mentioned above, PPI therapy use can potentially increase the risk of developing a *C. difficile* infection. Therefore, it should be used cautiously in high-risk patients for *C. difficile* [4]. Additionally, increasing evidence suggests a link between acid-suppression therapy and community- and hospital-acquired pneumonia [27]. Short-term PPI usage may increase the risk of community-acquired pneumonia compared to long-term users [4]. Several theories have been proposed to rationalize this association discussed previously. Initiating a PPI after the first case of pneumonia is associated with an increased risk of recurrent pneumonia. The risk seems to be elevated during the first 30 days of PPI use [27, 29].

Another potential side-effect of long-term PPI use is osteoporosis [4]. It is not recommended to discontinue a PPI in patients diagnosed with osteoporosis [4]. Additionally, concern for hip fractures and osteoporosis should not affect the decision to initiate PPIs for long-term use as long as other risk factors for osteoporosis are not present [4]. Patients treated with bisphosphonates such as alendronate should consider using H2RA for GERD as PPIs can potentially increase the risk of fracture for patients with osteoporosis by 38% [30]. While, all PPIs have similar safety profiles if a patient does experience a side effect with a particular PPI, switching to another PPI can potentially reduce adverse drug reactions [4].

Similar to H2RAs, drug interactions, while taking a PPI, can occur due to increasing the pH of the stomach [15]. Medications that require an acidic environment for absorption include itraconazole, ketoconazole, ampicillin, cephalosporins, sulfonylureas, dasatinib, iron salts, gefitinib, enteric-coated budesonide, and cyanocobalamin [31]. PPIs with specific antiretroviral agents such as atazanavir, delavirdine, and nelfinavir can decrease their bioavailability. Therefore, the coadministration of PPIs with these medications should be avoided [32].

Drug	Available formulation	Oral dose and frequency	Duration of use
Dexlansoprazole	Dual delayed-release oral capsule [34]	30 mg QD or 30 mg twice daily	4–8 weeks
Esomeprazole	Delayed-release oral capsule, delayed-release oral suspension, parenteral [37]	20 mg QD or 20 mg twice daily	4–8 weeks
Lansoprazole	Delayed-release oral capsule, delayed-release orally disintegrating tablets, oral powder [35]	15 mg QD or 15 mg twice daily	4–8 weeks
Omeprazole	Delayed-release capsules, delayed-release oral suspension, delayed-release orally disintegrating tablets, oral powder [38]	20 mg QD or 20 mg twice daily	4–8 weeks
Pantoprazole	delayed-release oral tablets, delayed-release oral suspension, parenteral [36]	20 mg QD or 20 mg twice daily	4–8 weeks
Rabeprazole	Delayed-release oral tablets [39]	20 mg QD or 20 mg twice daily	4–8 weeks

Table 3.
PPI dose, frequency, and duration of use recommended for GERD [34–39].

In 2009, the FDA issued warnings regarding concomitant PPI therapy and clopidogrel use. Clopidogrel is a prodrug activated to its active metabolite through the CYP 450 mechanism [4, 33]. All PPIs apart from dexlansoprazole have been found to exert some degree of CYP2C19 inhibition. Furthermore, all PPIs, including dexlansoprazole, are CYP2C19 substrates [33]. For a patient taking clopidogrel, PPIs can potentially reduce their antiplatelet effects due to CYP2C19 inhibition [4, 33]. Consider the use of a PPI with minimal or no impact on CYP2C19, such as rabeprazole, pantoprazole, lansoprazole, or dexlansoprazole if a PPI is necessary for a patient receiving clopidogrel as these did not result in a clinically significant reduction in exposure to the active metabolite of clopidogrel or clopidogrel-induced platelet inhibition [4, 33]. The use of omeprazole and esomeprazole significantly reduced the antiplatelet activity of clopidogrel when administered concomitantly or 12 hours apart [4, 33]. Pantoprazole is the preferred PPI in the hospital setting to minimize drug interactions as it is a weak CYP2C19 inhibitor (**Table 3**) [4, 33].

5. Non-acid suppressive therapy alternatives

5.1 Metoclopramide

The most commonly used prokinetic agent, metoclopramide, can be used to treat gastrointestinal motility disorders [40, 41]. Not only is metoclopramide a central dopamine D_2 receptor antagonist, but the medication also blocks the dopamine D_2 receptor in peripheral nerve endings and promotes the release of acetylcholine. This leads to increasing gastrointestinal motility, gastric emptying, and LES tone [40, 41].

Metoclopramide comes in oral and parenteral formulations for GERD use, with the dosing frequency summarized in **Table 4**. The onset of action for the oral formulation is 30–60 minutes, 1–3 minutes for intravenous, and 10–15 minutes for intramuscular injections [42, 43]. All formulations have a 1–2 hour duration with rapid

Formulation	Dosing	Duration
Oral	10–15 mg PO up to four times per day, 30 minutes before meals and at bedtime	Up to 12 weeks
Intravenous (IV)/ intramuscular (IM)	10 mg IV or IM up to four times per day, 30 minutes before meals and at bedtime	Up to 12 weeks

Table 4.
Dosing and duration of metoclopramide [42–44].

absorption [42, 43]. It is hepatically metabolized through oxidation, glucuronide, and sulfate conjugation [42, 43]. This results in the formation of monomethyl metoclopramide, which is an oxidative metabolite formed through CYP2D6 [42, 43].

Metoclopramide use is limited due to the central nervous system side effects such as agitation, irritability, depression, drowsiness, dystonic reactions, and tardive dyskinesia [45]. The most common side effects reported are dysgeusia, fatigue, restlessness, and drowsiness in more than 10% of patients taking metoclopramide. Severe side effects that may occur with metoclopramide are visual impairment, tardive dyskinesia, suicidal ideation, serotonin syndrome, seizures, porphyria, angioedema, and agranulocytosis [42, 43].

Metoclopramide should not be administered with atypical antipsychotics due to the increased risk of tardive dyskinesia, other extrapyramidal symptoms, and neuroleptic malignant syndrome [42, 43]. If atypical antipsychotics have to be used with this medication, patients must be monitored closely for movement disorders and CNS effects [42, 43]. Atypical antipsychotics should be discontinued upon first signs of dyskinesia [42, 43]. Due to the increased risk of tardive dyskinesia, treatment is not recommended beyond 12 weeks with metoclopramide use [44]. Populations with characteristics such as diabetes, geriatric, female, renal dysfunction, pediatric, or more than 12 weeks of metoclopramide use have all been associated with an increased risk of tardive dyskinesia and symptoms are often irreversible [42–44].

According to guidelines for the management of GERD, metoclopramide does not have a role in therapy unless gastroparesis is present [4]. Metoclopramide monotherapy is generally considered in patients refractory to conventional, acid-suppressive therapy [4]. Although PPIs are regarded as first-line, using a PPI alone is insufficient in approximately 30% of GERD patients [46, 47]. Prokinetic drugs have been used in clinical settings as a second-line option despite the fact that their benefits for GERD management are not well established [46, 47].

Although insufficient evidence is available regarding combination therapy with PPIs, the evidence for metoclopramide and H2RA combination therapy use did not show a clear benefit compared to monotherapy [4].

5.2 Baclofen

Baclofen is currently used off-label for GERD management. It works by stimulating the GABA-B receptor leading to reduced release of glutamate and aspartate and also reduces input into the alpha motor neurons [4]. Baclofen has been shown to reduce transient LES relaxation, reflux episodes, the number of postprandial acids and non-acid reflux events, nocturnal reflux activity, and belching attacks in two short-term randomized controlled trials [4]. Its use in GERD treatment is limited to patients refractory to PPI therapy and has no symptomatic relief [4].

Baclofen oral formulation onset of action is almost instantaneous; the medication is rapidly absorbed following administration [48, 49]. Dosing recommendations for refractory GERD patients is a trial of 5–20 mg given three times a day and must be dose-adjusted in CrCL < 80 ml/min since the kidney excretes 70–85% of baclofen as unchanged drug and metabolites [4, 48, 49].

Some limitations to baclofen use are the lack of long-term data as well as the side effects profile of the medication. Common side effects of baclofen include confusion, dizziness, drowsiness, headache, hypotonia, nausea, vomiting, and weakness [48, 49]. Severe side effects that may occur with baclofen are pulmonary embolism, renal failure, rhabdomyolysis, seizures, stroke, thrombosis, and ventricular tachycardia [48, 49].

Concurrent use of baclofen with opioid medications increases the risk of sedation and somnolence [48, 49]. Opioid medications for pain should be limited to patients who cannot tolerate alternative treatment options [48, 49]. Cough medications containing opioid medication should be avoided as well [48, 49].

5.3 Potassium-competitive acid blockers (P-CABs)

P-CABs have been developing for over the past 30 years [50]. Unlike PPIs, P-CABs directly inhibit gastric H^+/K^+-ATPase in a K^+-competitive, reversible manner and can bind to both the active and inactive forms of the ATPase pump resulting in a faster and longer duration of anti-secretory effect [26, 50]. Side effects of P-CABs include increased risk for gastric infection, obstruction of nutrient absorption, and increased levels of gastrin in the blood [50]. Advantages of P-CABs over PPIs have a faster onset of action with the maximum therapeutic effect observed in less than 2 hours post-administration [50]. P-CABs have a longer half-life compared to PPIs [50]. P-CABs have a better acid inhibitory effect than PPIs, and certain P-CABs have an effect that promotes gastric motility [50]. There are only three P-CABs available in Asia, with only one pending approval in the USA and Europe [50]. Revaprazan was the first-approved P-CAB in 2007 [50]. In South Korea and India, revaprazan is used to treat gastric ulcers, gastritis, and duodenal ulcers [50]. Revaprazan increases the percentage of time of pH > 4 in a dose-dependent manner [50]. In addition to suppressing acid, revaprazan has two more pharmacological effects: increased prostaglandin E2 and reduction in the production of leukotriene B4, which leads to gastroprotection [50]. However, the acid suppression ability and gastric pH > 4.0 holding time of revaprazan is not superior to conventional PPIs [26].

Vonoprazan fumarate has been approved in Japan since 2015 for treating gastroduodenal ulcers, healing and preventing erosive esophagitis, gastric protection in patients taking aspirin or NSAIDs, and eradicating *H. pylori* infection [50]. Vonoprazan can inhibit gastric proton pumps in neutral pH, unlike PPIs that need to be activated by an acidic environment [50]. It can be taken without regard to meals [50]. Vonoprazan is currently under phase III trial in the USA and Europe [50]. In healing erosive esophagitis, vonoprazan 20 mg compared to lansoprazole 30 mg showed similar results in healing when compared to lansoprazole [50]. In patients with non-erosive reflux disease, vonoprazan was studied at doses of 10 and 20 mg compared to placebo. Patients experienced less severe GERD symptoms with vonoprazan compared to placebo [50]. Safety concerns about the long-term use of vonoprazan have been raised because of the significant elevation of serum gastrin levels compared with conventional PPI therapy [26]. Increased incidence of gastric endocrine cell tumors in a nonclinical carcinogenicity study has been correlated with the increased serum gastrin level, but the impact on humans is still unknown [26].

Tegoprazan has been approved and available since July 2018 in South Korea for treating erosive esophagitis and non-erosive reflux disease [50]. In patients with erosive esophagitis, tegoprazan (50 or 100 mg) was compared to esomeprazole 40 mg for 8 weeks [50]. Results showed that both doses of tegoprazan were non-inferior [50]. Although not currently available in the United States, P-CABs may play a role in GERD management soon after FDA approval.

6. GERD treatment in special populations: Pregnancy

Pregnancy is considered a likely risk factor in GERD, with approximately 80% of pregnant women, in their third-trimester experiencing what is known as gestational reflux [51, 52]. This increased prevalence of gestational reflux is likely due to decreased LES pressure [51]. Heartburn and nausea may be expected in a healthy pregnancy, but there are concerns over specific agents used in treatment [51]. Treatment for gestational reflux calls for "step-up" therapy, starting with lifestyle modifications or alternative medicines such as acupuncture [51]. If that fails to provide enough relief, the following options would be antacids, sucralfate, or metoclopramide [51]. A step up from these regimens, if deemed ineffective, would be H2RAs, and a step up from that would be PPIs [51]. The American College of Gastroenterology (ACG) GERD guidelines do not have an extensive algorithm for gestational reflux [4]. The guidelines mention that sucralfate does not have a role in non-pregnant GERD patients, and PPIs are safe in pregnant patients if clinically indicated [4].

The FDA classified drugs for pregnancy in categories that help define a drug's potential risk of fetal harm [51]. Category A of the FDA's classification means that there are well-controlled studies in humans, and the drug shows no fetal risk [51]. None of the pharmacological options of therapy for gestational reflux are considered Category A [51]. Category B means that animal studies show no risks, but human studies do now show adequate evidence expressing safety [51]. All H2RA's, sucralfate, metoclopramide, and most PPIs except for omeprazole are Category B [51]. Category C shows that animal studies show risk, but human studies lack the evidence to support safety [51]. Omeprazole and cisapride are considered Category C drugs [51]. As for all of the antacids that are aluminum, calcium, or magnesium-containing, those fall under Category N by the FDA [51]. Category N is defined as no classification [51].

Following the step-up treatment guideline, lifestyle modifications such as eating smaller meals, not eating at night, elevating the head of the bed, and avoiding postural changes and dietary triggers are considered the first line [51]. Next on the step-up is antacids, sucralfate, or metoclopramide which are mostly considered safe with a few exceptions [51]. One exception is magnesium trisilicate which is not recommended long term [51]. Long-term use of magnesium trisilicate has been associated with nephrolithiasis, hypotonia, cardiovascular impairment, and respiratory disease in the fetus [51]. It is also recommended that pregnant women avoid sodium bicarbonate as it can cause fluid overload and metabolic alkalosis [51]. Sucralfate is Category B and is generally regarded as acceptable for use [51]. Metoclopramide is a promotility agent that is part of the step-up therapy for pregnant women. Another promotility agent is cisapride which has shown evidence of being embryotoxic and fetotoxic in animals, and the FDA has removed this drug for causing fatal cardiac arrhythmias [51]. H2RAs are generally safe for pregnancy, except for nizatidine [51]. Nizatidine has been known to cause spontaneous abortion, congenital malformations, low birth weight, and fewer live births have been reported in animal studies [51]. Ranitidine was the only H2RA whose efficacy during pregnancy has been established, but it has recently been removed from the market for having a carcinogenic metabolite NDMA [51]. Next on the step-up therapy is PPIs which are generally safe for use in pregnancy except for omeprazole [51]. Omeprazole is embryotoxic and fetotoxic in animals, and case reports in humans show similar concerns [51].

7. Special populations: Elderly

Management of GERD in the elderly is generally similar to the adult population. However, there are specific concerns regarding treatments in the geriatric population. Most elderly patients have co-morbid conditions such as cardiovascular disease, hypertension, depression, and osteoporosis that require multiple medications [53]. Many medicines to treat these conditions can lead to decreased LES pressure, esophageal motility, and direct esophageal injury [53]. Examples include calcium channel blockers, benzodiazepines, nitrates, nonsteroidal anti-inflammatory drugs, and anticholinergic agents [53]. Aggressive, individualized treatments may be warranted due to the high risk of complications from GERD and co-morbid illnesses in this patient population [54]. Motility agents may improve LES tone, although success is limited in patients with severe disease [53]. Higher doses, up to four times daily, of H2RA may be required in some elderly patients for adequate acid suppression and symptom relief; however, proper dose adjustment is needed if patients have renal insufficiency [53]. As with most medications, the side effect, and drug interaction profile could be more pronounced in the geriatric population. No evidence-based guidelines support specific treatment options in those over 65. However, PPIs are usually first-line medical therapy in patients with GERD [54]. PPIs provide excellent acid suppression. Capsules may be opened and sprinkled in water, juice, or applesauce. Besides, lansoprazole and omeprazole are available in powder formulation for those that have difficulty or are unable to swallow [53]. Maintenance therapy is usually required in this population as long-term treatment is necessary to prevent relapse. Of note, unless the patient is high-risk (e.g., Barrett esophagitis, erosive esophagitis, chronic NSAID use, etc.), the Beers criteria advises against using PPIs continuously for > 8 weeks for patients ≥65 due to the risk of *Clostridium difficile* infection and bone loss [55]. Beers criteria also suggests avoiding H2RA use in patients who have delirium [55].

Effects of prolonged acid suppression can include: reduced absorption of nutrients, osteoporosis, and drug metabolism interference [53]. Although these effects are controversial, monitoring patients on long-term acid-suppressive therapy is still important. Surgery may be warranted in those with dysplasia, esophageal adenocarcinoma, and Barrett's esophagus [54]. There are important factors to consider regarding the treatment and management of the elderly compared to the younger population. However, with appropriate direction, GERD can be treated in most elderly patients with successful outcomes.

8. Conclusion

GERD can be managed with pharmacological and non-pharmacological options. Treatment options should be individualized based on presenting factors. If poorly or not treated, it can lead to complications such as esophageal cancer, erosive esophagitis, Barrett's esophagus, and possible bleeding and scarring. Routine follow-ups should be completed to ensure adherence and medication effectiveness. PPIs should be used as first-line therapy for treating and managing GERD, along with patient education on lifestyle modifications. Other pharmacotherapy regimens should be explored if shown ineffective, or surgical interventions may be required.

Author details

Anthony Wilks[1,2], Ladan Panahi[1,2]*, George Udeani[1,2] and Salim Surani[1,2,3,4]

1 Department of Pharmacy Practice, Texas A&M Rangel College of Pharmacy, Kingsville, TX, USA

2 Department of Pharmacy Practice, Texas A&M Rangel College of Pharmacy, College Station, TX, USA

3 Section of Pulmonary—Critical Care and Fellowship Program, Corpus Christi Medical Center, Corpus Christi, TX, USA

4 Department of Medicine, College of Medicine, Texas A&M University, College Station, TX, USA

*Address all correspondence to: panahi@tamu.edu

References

[1] Locke R. The Prevalence and Impact of Gastroesophageal Reflux Disease. n.d. Available from: https://www.aboutgerd.org/prevalence.html. [Retrieved: 18 January 2021]

[2] Clarrett DM, Hachem C. Gastroesophageal reflux disease (GERD). Missouri Medicine. 2018;**115**(3):214

[3] De Giorgi F, Palmiero M, Esposito I, Mosca F, Cuomo R. Pathophysiology of gastro-oesophageal reflux disease. Acta Otorhinolaryngologica Italica. 2006;**26**(5):241

[4] Katz PO, Gerson LB, Vela MF. Guidelines for the diagnosis and management of gastroesophageal reflux disease. American Journal of Gastroenterology - ACG. 2013;**108**(3):308

[5] Scholten T. Long-term management of gastroesophageal reflux disease with pantoprazole. Therapeutics and Clinical Risk Management. 2007;**3**(2):231

[6] Gelhot AR, Scott M. Gastroesophageal reflux disease: Diagnosis and management. American Family Physician. 1999;**59**(5):1161

[7] Kang J-E, Kang J. Lifestyle measures in the management of gastro-oesophageal reflux disease: Clinical and pathophysiological considerations. Therapeutic Advances in Chronic Disease. 2015;**6**(2):51-64

[8] Smith L. Updated ACG Guidelines for Diagnosis and Treatment of GERD. 2005. Available from: https://www.aafp.org/afp/2005/0615/p2376.html [Retrieved: 18 January 2021]

[9] Salisbury BH, Terrell JM. Antacids. StatPearls; 2020 [Internet]

[10] Aluminum Hydroxide, Magnesium Hydroxide, Simethicone Chewable Tablet—Aluminum Hydroxide, Magnesium Trisilicate Chewable Tablet—Bisacodyl Oral Tablet—Bismuth Subcitrate Potassium, Metronidazole, Tetracycline Hydrochloride Oral Capsule—Calcium Carbonate Oral Tablet—Calcium Carbonate, Magnesium Hydroxide Chewable Tablet—Prednisone Oral Tablet. Interactions. Clinical Pharmacology [Internet]. Tampa, FL: Elsevier; 2021. Available from: http://www.clinicalpharmacology.com. [Cited: 21 January 2021]

[11] Mag-Al-Plus XS. Magnesium Hydroxide, Aluminum Hydroxide and Dimethicone Suspension Package Insert. Greenville, SC: Pharmaceutical Associates Inc.; 2019

[12] Tzanakis IP, Papadaki AN, Wei M, et al. Magnesium carbonate for phosphate control in patients on hemodialysis. A randomized controlled trial. International Urology and Nephrology. 2008;**40**(1):193-201

[13] Antunes C et al. Gastroesophageal Reflux Disease. National Institutes of Health; 2020 [Internet]

[14] Braunstein LZ, Kantor ED, O'Connell K, et al. Analysis of ranitidine-associated N-nitrosodimethylamine production under simulated physiologic conditions. JAMA Network Open. 2021;**4**(1):e2034766

[15] Nugent CC, Terrell JM. H2 Blockers. National Institutes of Health; 2020 [Internet]

[16] Gyawali CP, Fass R. Management of gastroesophageal reflux disease. Gastroenterology. 2018;**154**(2):302-318

[17] Cantú TG, Korek JS. Central nervous system reactions to histamine-2 receptor blockers. Annals of Internal Medicine. 1991;**114**(12):1027-1034

[18] McGuigan JE. A consideration of the adverse effects of cimetidine. Gastroenterology. 1981;**80**(1):181-192

[19] Tleyjeh IM, Abdulhak AAB, Riaz M, et al. The association between histamine 2 receptor antagonist use and *Clostridium difficile* infection: A systematic review and meta-analysis. PLoS One. 2013;**8**(3):e56498

[20] Laheij RJ, Sturkenboom MC, Hassing R-J, Dieleman J, Stricker BH, Jansen JB. Risk of community-acquired pneumonia and use of gastric acid-suppressive drugs. Journal of the American Medical Association. 2004;**292**(16):1955-1960

[21] Anderson WD, Strayer SM, et al. Common questions about the management of gastroesophageal reflux disease. American Family Physician. 2015;**91**(10):692-697

[22] Scarpignato C, Gatta L, Zullo A, Blandizzi C. Effective and safe proton pump inhibitor therapy in acid-related diseases—A position paper addressing benefits and potential harms of acid suppression. BMC Medicine. 2016;**14**(1):1-35

[23] Gąsiorowska A. The role of pH in symptomatic relief and effective treatment of gastroesophageal reflux disease. Przeglad Gastroenterologiczny. 2017;**12**(4):244

[24] Shin JM, Sachs G. Pharmacology of proton pump inhibitors. Current Gastroenterology Reports. 2008;**10**(6):528-534

[25] Howden CW. Update on dual delayed-release PPI formulations. Gastroenterology & Hepatology. 2010;**6**(7):417

[26] Kim DK, Lee K-H, Kim S-J, et al. Effects of tegoprazan, a novel potassium-competitive acid blocker, on rat models of gastric acid-related disease. The Journal of Pharmacology and Experimental Therapeutics. 2019;**369**(3):318-327

[27] Eurich DT, Sadowski CA, Simpson SH, Marrie TJ, Majumdar SR. Recurrent community-acquired pneumonia in patients starting acid-suppressing drugs. The American Journal of Medicine. 2010;**123**(1):47-53

[28] Ali T, Roberts DN, Tierney WM. Long-term safety concerns with proton pump inhibitors. The American Journal of Medicine. 2009;**122**(10):896-903

[29] Sarkar M, Hennessy S, Yang Y-X. Proton-pump inhibitor use and the risk for community-acquired pneumonia. Annals of Internal Medicine. 2008;**149**(6):391-398

[30] Jaynes M, Kumar AB. The risks of long-term use of proton pump inhibitors: A critical review. Therapeutic Advances in Drug Safety. 2019;**10**:2042

[31] Hirschowitz B, Worthington J, Mohnen J. Vitamin B12 deficiency in hypersecretors during long-term acid suppression with proton pump inhibitors. Alimentary Pharmacology & Therapeutics. 2008;**27**(11):1110-1121

[32] Fang AF, Damle BD, LaBadie RR, Crownover PH, Hewlett D Jr, Glue PW. Significant decrease in nelfinavir systemic exposure after omeprazole coadministration in healthy subjects. Pharmacotherapy: The Journal of Human Pharmacology and Drug Therapy. 2008;**28**(1):42-50

[33] Kinoshita Y, Ishimura N, Ishihara S. Advantages and disadvantages of long-term proton pump inhibitor use. Journal of Neurogastroenterology and Motility. 2018;**24**(2):182

[34] Takeda Pharmaceuticals America. Dexilant (Dexlansoprazole) Package Insert. Deerfield, IL: Takeda Pharmaceuticals America, Inc.; 2020

[35] Takeda Pharmaceuticals America. Prevacid (Lansoprazole) Capsules, Tablets Package Insert. Deerfield, IL: Takeda Pharmaceuticals America, Inc.; 2020

[36] Wyeth Pharmaceuticals. Protonix (Pantoprazole) Package Insert. Philadelphia, PA: Wyeth Pharmaceuticals; 2020

[37] AstraZeneca. Nexium (Esomeprazole) Capsules, Granules Package Insert. Wilmington, DE: AstraZeneca; 2020

[38] AstraZeneca. Prilosec (Omeprazole) Package Insert. Wilmington, DE: AstraZeneca; 2020

[39] Eisai Inc. Aciphex (Rabeprazole) Delayed-Release Tablets Package Insert. Woodcliff Lake, NJ: Eisai Inc; 2020

[40] Dilawari J, Misiewicz J. Action of oral metoclopramide on the gastrooesophageal junction in man. Gut. 1973;**14**(5):380-382

[41] Howard F, Sharp D. Effect of metoclopramide on gastric emptying during labour. British Medical Journal. 1973;**1**(5851):446-448

[42] Ani Pharmaceuticals. Metoclopramide Hydrochloride Oral Solution Package Insert. Baudette, MN: Ani Pharmaceuticals; 2019

[43] Salix Pharmaceuticals IF. Metozolv ODT (Metoclopramide Hydrochloride) Orally Disintegrating Tablet Package Insert. Raleigh: Salix Pharmaceuticals; 2019

[44] Ani Pharmaceuticals. Reglan (Metoclopramide) Oral Tablet Package Insert. Baudette, MN: Ani Pharmaceuticals; 2020

[45] Rao A, Camilleri M. Metoclopramide and tardive dyskinesia. Alimentary Pharmacology & Therapeutics. 2010;**31**(1):11-19

[46] Miwa H, Inoue K, Ashida K, et al. Randomised clinical trial: Efficacy of the addition of a prokinetic, mosapride citrate, to omeprazole in the treatment of patients with non-erosive reflux disease—A double-blind, placebo-controlled study. Alimentary Pharmacology & Therapeutics. 2011;**33**(3):323-332

[47] Hsu YC, Yang TH, Hsu WL, et al. Mosapride as an adjunct to lansoprazole for symptom relief of reflux oesophagitis. British Journal of Clinical Pharmacology. 2010;**70**(2):171-179

[48] Metacel Pharmaceuticals, LLC. Ozobax (Baclofen) Oral Solution Package Insert. Athens, GA: Metacel Pharmaceuticals, LLC; 2010

[49] Northstar Rx LLC. Baclofen Tablet [Prescribing Information]. Memphis, TN: Northstar Rx LLC; 2019

[50] Shibli F, Kitayama Y, Fass R. Novel therapies for gastroesophageal reflux disease: Beyond proton pump inhibitors. Current Gastroenterology Reports. 2020;**22**(4):1-13

[51] Thélin CS, Richter JE. The management of heartburn during pregnancy and lactation. Alimentary Pharmacology & Therapeutics. 2020;**51**(4):421-434

[52] Kellerman R, Kintanar T. Gastroesophageal reflux disease. Primary Care; Clinics in Office Practice. 2017;**44**(4):561-573

[53] Chait MM. Gastroesophageal reflux disease: Important considerations for the older patients. World Journal of Gastrointestinal Endoscopy. 2010;**2**(12):388

[54] Bacak BS, Patel M, Tweed E, Danis P. What is the best way to manage GERD symptoms in the elderly? J Fam Pract. 2006;**55**(3):251-258

[55] By the American Geriatrics Society Beers Criteria Update Expert Panel. American Geriatrics Society 2019 updated AGS Beers Criteria(R) for potentially inappropriate medication use in older adults. Journal of the American Geriatrics Society. 2019;**67**(4):674-694

Chapter 5

The Role of Proton Pump Inhibitors in the Treatment of Barrett's Esophagus

Zaim Gashi, Arjeta Gashi and Fadil Sherifi

Abstract

Barrett's esophagus (BE), as a more frequent complication of gastroesophageal reflux disease, is a metaplastic condition in which the normal squamous epithelium of the esophagus is replaced by specialized intestinal metaplastic epithelium, and that, in about 10% of patients with gastroesophageal reflux disease (GERD) and the main condition for dysplasia and adenocarcinoma. The incidence of adenocarcinoma of the cardia is rapidly increasing at a rate that exceeds that of any other cancer. Recently, acid suppression with proton pump inhibitors (PPIs) has become the cornerstone of treatment for patients with BE. Many worldwide investigations showed that PPI is effective in the regression of BE with low-grade dysplasia and especially for the regression of intestinal metaplasia, incomplete or complete, for long-term use of these medicaments. This chapter reviews the specific endpoints of such treatment, included and our results for this dilemma.

Keywords: Barrett's esophagus, low-grade dysplasia, proton pump inhibitor, regression, gastroesophageal reflux disease (GERD)

1. Introduction

Gastroesophageal reflux disease (GERD) is accepted as a cornerstone etiological factor for Barrett's esophagus (BE), which is a major predisposition to esophageal adenocarcinoma.

GERD is a precursor to BE, which represents intestinal metaplasia (IM), [1] and the latter is most likely a precursor to esophageal cancer. Progression from Barrett's to dysplasia is estimated to be in about 20% of cases [2]. Chronic heartburn can progress to Barrett's, so EGD (esophagogastroduodenoscopy) is recommended every 5 years for these cases, but also for cases taking medication for chronic GERD [3].

BE is a condition in which there is an abnormal change (metaplastic tissue) with the replacement of multilayered epithelial cells, under the long-term influence of gastroesophageal reflux, with specialized intestinal cells that are present only in the small and large intestines. This change is considered to be a precursor of distal malignancy of the esophagus as it is associated with a high incidence of further transition to adenocarcinoma of the esophagus, with a highly malignant nature [1, 2].

BE is diagnosed with endoscopy: we encounter inflammatory, erosive, ulcerative changes up to narrowing of the distal lumen of the esophagus, classified according to

Los Angeles A-D, followed by microscopic examination of the tissue from the affected area from the biopsies obtained. BE cells are classified into four categories: nondysplastic (such as incomplete and complete intestinal metaplasia), low-grade dysplasia, high-grade dysplasia, and carcinoma.

Up to the level of low dysplasia, the changes can be treated with PPI, including here the fundoplication according to Nissen. High-grade dysplasia and early stages of adenocarcinoma can be treated with endoscopic resection or radiofrequency ablation [1]. Later stages of adenocarcinoma can be treated by surgical resection. Nondysplastic or low-grade (LGD) cases are managed by annual surveillance with endoscopy or treatment with radiofrequency ablation. It should be borne in mind that in cases with high-grade dysplasia (HGD), the risk of developing cancer can be 10% per patient-year or more, so treatment is needed as soon as possible [4].

A greater extent of dysplasia has a significantly higher risk of cancer as well as the presence of an endoscopic abnormality [5].

BE is thought to be an adaptation to the chronic exposure of acid reflux, but also of another nature, in the esophagus for a long time [6].

2. Pathophysiology

BE reflects chronic chemical inflammation, as a consequence of persistent gastroesophageal reflux. Basically, it is the acidic content of the stomach, bile and small intestines, and pancreas as a potential cause of reflux changes. From this reflux, different cells react, including stem cells that express HOXA13, which are characterized by distal (intestinal) characteristics and compete with normal squamous cells [7].

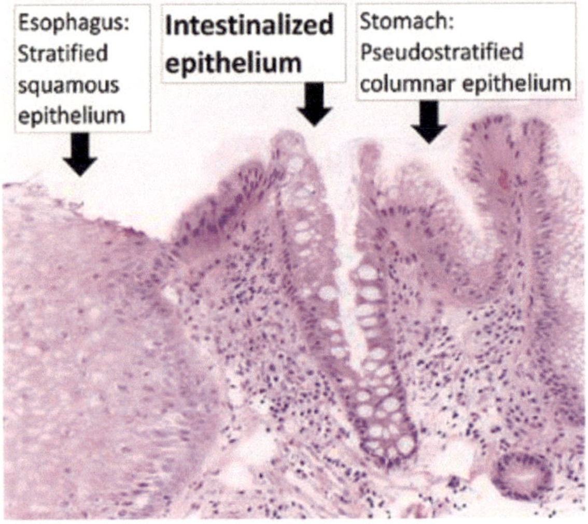

Figure 1.
Histopathology of Barrett's esophagus, showing intestinalized epithelium with goblet cells, as opposed to normal stratified squamous epithelium of the esophagus, and pseudostratified columnar epithelium of the fundus of the stomach. The submucosa displays an infiltrate including lymphocytes and plasma cells, constituting an underlying chronic inflammation. The area between the stratified and the intestinalized epithelium displays reactive changes, but there is no secondary dysplasia in this case. H&E stain [11].

This explains the participation of HER2/neu (also called ERBB2) and overexpressed (lineage-dependent) cancer cells during the process of carcinogenesis, and the efficacy of targeted therapy against the Her-2 receptor with Trastuzumab (Herceptin) in the treatment of adenocarcinomas in the gastroesophageal junction.

It cannot be determined which of the patients with reflux will develop BE later. While chronic heartburn affects the development of BE, researchers have not observed a strong association between the severity of reflux and the development of BE. But there was also the phenomenon that people with BE have no symptoms of heartburn at all.

Patients with bulimia, an eating disorder, are more likely to develop BE because bulimia can cause severe acid reflux and because it damages the epithelial cells in the esophagus to a large extent, disrupting the so-called "tight junction." between the mucous cells [8, 9].

The very act of bile acids entering the esophagus can be an important factor in carcinogenesis [10]. Chronic patients with GERD and BE are exposed to high concentrations of deoxycholic acid, which has cytotoxic effects and can cause DNA damage (**Figure 1**) [12, 13].

3. Diagnosis

For the diagnosis of GERD and BE, in addition to the relevant clinical data, the macroscopic view during the endoscopy and the microscopic examination after biopsies have been taken are also necessary. In non-dysplastic Barrett's, goblet cells and specialized intestinal cells are characteristic, which have replaced the previous multilayered epithelium. Of course, this is the body's initial protective reaction to the reflux content, but it does not withstand time, following BE with a tendency to fail to turn into adenocarcinoma (**Figures 2** and **3**).

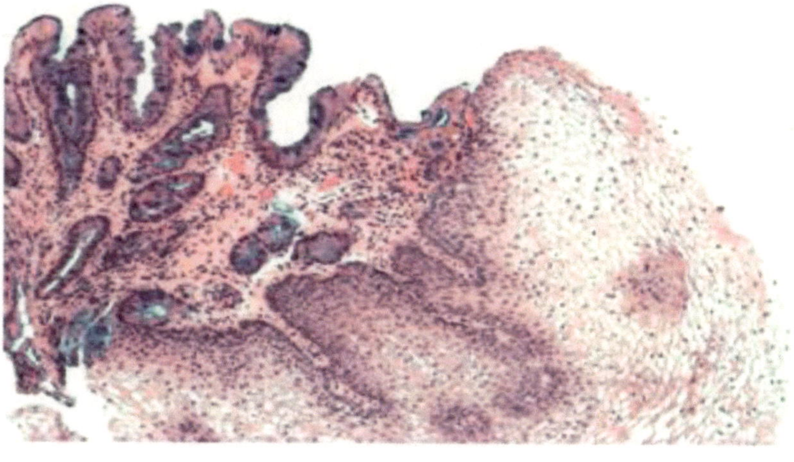

Figure 2.
Micrograph showing Barrett's esophagus – Columnar epithelia with goblet cells – On the left side of image; and normal stratified squamous epithelium on the right side of image Alcian blue stain [11].

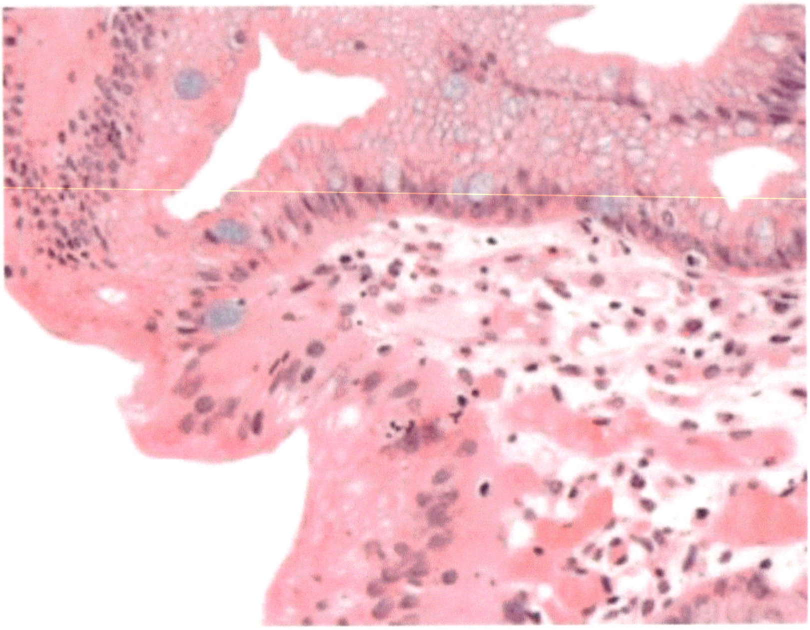

Figure 3.
High-magnification micrograph of Barrett's esophagus showing the characteristic goblet cells, Alcian blue stain [11].

4. Management

BE is not always associated with dysplasia. According to the latest recommendations, if a patient with BE is diagnosed and if the last two endoscopic examinations with biopsy have confirmed the absence of dysplasia, then the patient should have the next endoscopy within 3 years [3, 10, 14].

The risk of malignancy is highest in the United States in Caucasian men over 50 years of age with more than 5 years of symptoms. Although watchful waiting is preferred in cases of BE, for cases with dysplasia, balloon-based radiofrequency ablation, invented by Ganz, Stern, and Zelickson in 1999, is a new treatment modality for the treatment of BE and dysplasia and has been the subject of numerous published clinical trials. The findings demonstrate radiofrequency ablation has an efficacy of 90% or greater with respect to complete clearance of BE and dysplasia with the durability of up to 5 years and a favorable safety profile [15–18].

The results of antireflux surgery, specifically fundoplication, have not been proven to prevent esophageal cancer. Proton pump inhibitors have been shown to be effective in limiting the progression of esophageal cancer. Laser treatment is used in severe dysplasia, while open malignancy may require surgery, radiation therapy, or systemic chemotherapy. A recent 5-year study randomly showed that photodynamic therapy using photofrin is statistically more effective in eliminating dysplastic foci than the use of a proton pump inhibitor alone [19].

The heterogeneous nature of Barrett's explains the wide spectrum of the degree of mutational overlap between adjacent BE and eopphageal adenocarcinoma [20].

Anti-reflux surgery (ARS), namely laparoscopic fundoplication, is the last step in GERD management. Its objectives are LES, basal pressure increase and hiatal repair [21].

Recent studies show that nonsteroidal anti-inflammatory drugs (NSAIDS), such as aspirin, have shown evidence of preventing esophageal cancer in people with BE [22, 23]. However, none of these studies have provided reliable evidence for the effect of these drugs in the prevention of esophageal adenocarcinoma in the field of BE.

BE is thought to be the result of esophageal epithelium in response to damage. The development of BE is a consequence of long-term GERD. Barrett's epithelium, due to its specific histological features, can be expected to be more resistant to aggressive acidic stomach contents. Diagnosis of Barrett's patients always requires histological confirmation to allow better monitoring of patients, according to the degree of change in Barrett's patients.

HP type	N	%
IM	40	80.0
LGD	10	20.0
HGD	—	—
Total	50	100.0

Legend: HP – histopathologic type, IM – intestinal metaplasia, LGD - low grade dysplasia, HGD – high grade dysplasia.

Table 1.
Structure of patients with BE at the beginning of the study.

	IM		LGD		HGD	
	N	%	N	%	N	%
IM	20	50.0	2	20.0	—	—
LGD	4	10.0	5	50.0	—	—
HGD	—	—	—	—	—	—
NERD	16	40.0	3	30.0	—	—
Total	40	100.0	10	100.0	—	—

Table 2.
Evaluation of patients with BE after 2 years of treatment.

Evaluation	SSBE		LSBE		TOTAL	
	N	%	N	%	N	%
Regression	17	43.6	4	36.4	21	42.0
Stable	21	53.8	4	36.4	25	50.0
Progression	1	2.6	3	27.3	4	8.0
Total	39	100.0	11	100.0	50	100.0
Progression/Other	Z = -2.66, P = 0.0078					

SSBE: Dmax = 0.32 > D (39,0.05) = 0.22 and P < 0.05.
Dmax = 0.32 > D (39;0.01) = 0.26 and P < 0.01.
LSBE: Dmax = 0.06 < D (11;0.05) = 0.391 and P > 0.05.

Table 3.
Evaluation of patients with BE by endoscopic type.

The PPI class is the most potent type of acid suppression therapy. PPIs are replaced by benzimidazoles that continuously bind H + K + ATP as the final step in gastric acid secretion. Group members include omeprazole, lansoprazole, pantoprazole, rabeprazole, and esomeprazole. Standard doses of each type of drug may have a similar inhibitory effect. Omeprazole is the longest documented agent, while newer agents, rabeprazole and pantoprazole, have less interaction than both with the cytochrome P450 metabolism. Several studies have shown the superiority of PPI over H2RAs in the treatment of reflux esophagitis.

Of the 50 patients with BE according to histopathological type, 40 or 80.0% were IM, 10 or 20% were LGD and there was no case of HGD (**Table 1**).

Out of the 40 IM patients included in our study, after 2 years of treatment, only 20 patients or 50.0% had IM, 4 or 10.0% had LGD and 16 patients or 40.0% had NERD. Of the 10 patients with LGD after 2 years of treatment, only 5 patients or 50.0% had LGD, 2 patients or 20.0% had IM, and 3 patients or 30.0% had NERD (non-erosive reflux disease) (**Table 2**).

Patients of the endoscopic type Long segment of Barrett's esophagus (LSBE) have a more frequent progression of 27.3% compared with 2.6% to patients of the endoscopic type Short Segment of Barrett's esophagus (SSBE) 2.6% difference with significant statistical significance ($Z = -2.66$, $P = 0.0078$), (**Table 3**).

With the Kolmogar-Smirn test, we confirmed a statistically significant difference in the regressions of changes in BE, when we have to do with SSBE ($P < 0.05$ and 0.01), but also not a significant difference in the evolution of changes in BE, progression, or regression, when we have to do with LSBE ($P > 0.05$) (**Figure 4**).

The correlation of histopathological type and disease regression in patients with BE, in our study, did not result in a significant difference (Fisher Exact test, $P = 0.487$). From the group with intestinal metaplasia, 40.0% of patients and 50.0% of patients in the LGD (low-grade dysplasia) group had regression (**Figure 5**, **Table 4**).

Of the 70 patients with GERD regression, we had 40 or 57.1%, and of the 50 patients with BE regression we had 21 or 42.0% difference without any statistically significant value ($P = 0.138$), 34.3% of patients with GERD was stable and 50.0% of patients with BE without significant difference ($P = 0.05$), and we had progression in

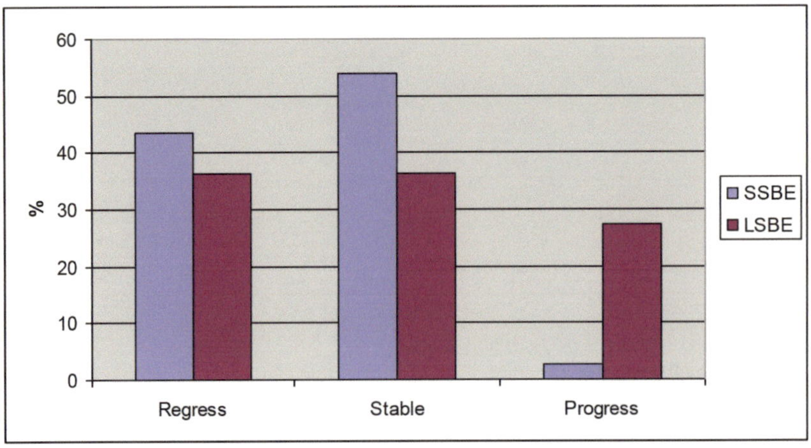

Figure 4.
Regression in patients with BE by endoscopic type [24].

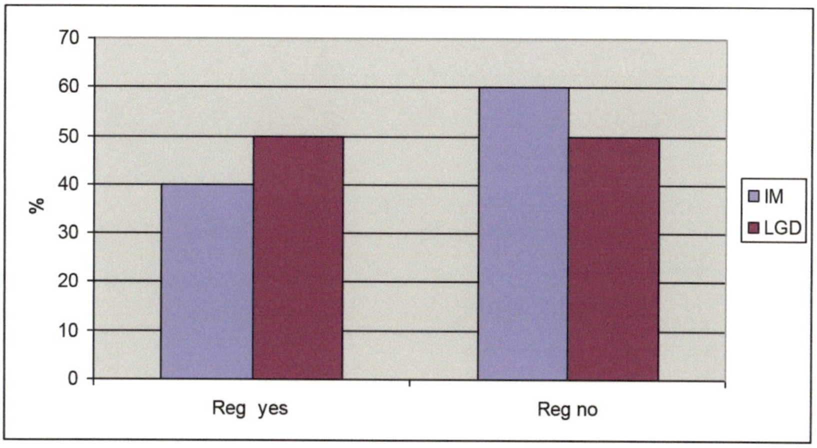

Figure 5.
Regression in patients with BE by histopathological type [24].

Types of HP		Regression		Total
		Yes	No	
IM	N	16	24	40
	%	40.0	60.0	100.0
LGD	N	5	5	10
	%	50.0	50.0	100.0
Total	N	21	29	50
	%	42.0	58.0	100.0
Fisher Exact Test		P = 0.487		

Table 4.
Regression among patients with BE according to histopathological type.

8.6% of patients with GERD and 8.0% of patients with BE without significant difference (P = 1.00).

Also with the Fisher test, we did not get a significant difference between the groups (P = 1.00) according to the degree of progression.

However, there is a significant intra-group difference between the two groups, where patients with regression and stable changes after IPP treatment visibly dominate over those with progression. The test was performed with the Colmogar-Smirn test for one sample.

After treatment of patients with PPI, there was more regression of the disease in patients with GERD than in those with BE (**Table 5**).

4.1 Progression of erosive esophagitis to BE

Eighty-three patients (54% male, median age 59 years) with mild esophagitis were treated with continuous PPIs and cisapride at doses sufficient to control symptoms (**Table 3**) [25]. After 2 years, during the second "follow-up" endoscopy, 12 (15%) had developed BE histologically confirmed in the biopsies taken. Of these patients, nine

Evaluation	GERD		BE		Fisher test
	N	%	N	%	
Regression	40	57.1	21	42.0	$P = 0.138$
Stable	24	34.3	25	50.0	$P = 0.09$
Progression	6	8.6	4	8.0	$P = 1.00$
Total	70	100.0	50	100.0	
Fisher test Progression/Other		P = 1.00			

GERD: Dmax = 0.25 > D (70:0.05) = 0.16 and P < 0.05.
Dmax = 0.25 > D (70:0.01) = 0.19 and P < 0.01.
BE: Dmax = 0.26 > D (50:0.05) = 0.19 and P < 0.05.
Dmax = 0.26 > D (50:0.01) = 0.23 and P < 0.01.

Table 5.
Comparison of the effect after PPI treatment of patients with BE and GERD.

had short-segment disease (SSBE<3 cm) and the other three had long-segment BE (LSBE>3 cm).

Of great importance was the development of lower esophageal sphincter pressures (LOSPs) patients who developed BE, had significantly reduced LOSP compared to those who had not progressed, but their age and gender were not stated.

In another study by Isolauri et al. [26] 6 (or 12%) of 50 medically treated patients with GERD symptoms and abnormal pH values developed BE, defined as the presence of epithelial specialized columnar-intestinal histologically confirmed at least 3 cm. over the most proximal gastric fold, during a follow-up period of 17–22 years. Four of these patients had grade I esophagitis and two grade II esophagitis at index endoscopy (Savary-Miller classification). In this study, the distinguishing characteristics between those who developed and those who did not develop BE were not given. In an international, multicenter study of the use of maintenance omeprazole in patients with reflux esophagitis who were refractory to long-term histamine 2 receptor antagonist (H2RA) therapy, 20 of 166 patients (12%) developed BE during a median follow-up of 6.5 years (range: 1.4–11.2) [27]. All patients were taking omeprazole at all times, but dosage and demographic characteristics were not stated.

The study by McDougall et al. reported that 3 of 33 (9%) patients presenting with esophagitis developed BE, during a follow-up period of up to 4.5 years [28]. In terms of gender, all three patients were male. It was reported that a patient with minimal esophagitis and a small hiatus hernia at index endoscopy developed a 5-cm length of BE. But, from the anamnestic data, this patient was taking ranitidine 150 mg twice a day. Another patient had grade III esophagitis initially, which reverted to grade I at 2 months of H2RA but then developed a 5-cm segment of BE. This patient was also taking ranitidine 150 mg twice daily. The third patient with grade III esophagitis initially developed a 6 cm BE at his fourth endoscopy 18 months later, although this patient was started on omeprazole 20 mg daily after 12 months but despite this, BE was diagnosed.

In another study, patients with reflux esophagitis cured after PPI treatment continued with the maintenance dose for 14.6 months. Repeated endoscopy was repeated in those patients who had repeated symptoms [1]. Two patients developed BE; one of class II (Savary-Miller classification) after 24 months of follow-up and one of class III after 8 months. In this study, the length of BE and the fact which criteria were used for the diagnosis of BE are not given. These patients were part of a study of 692 patients with GERD, where more than half of the patients had esophageal reflux, but it is not known which ones underwent endoscopy, nor the demographic details of those with BE and those without this pathology. The authors in a retrospective analysis of 582 patients with grade I-III esophagitis (Savary-Monnier classification) diagnosed at endoscopy during a 27-year period, in the follow-up for 6.5 years, 45 (8%) developed BE [29]. But the study was reported only in abstract form and neither the diagnostic criteria, the demographic characteristics of the patients, nor the drug history were described.

In an interesting study investigating the progression of NERD in BE, Bajbouj et al. [30] described that two of a group of 34 patients (6%) with typical GERD symptoms and a normal endoscopy had developed BE after a 35-month follow-up. No data are given for the treatment. As in many other works, the length of the BE segment, as well as the demographic data for the patients, were not given. As stated above, from 1–13% of patients with erosive esophagitis develop BE each year.

4.2 Indirect evidence of progression

El-Serag and Sonnenberg reported the relationship between the middle forms of erosive oesophagitis, esophageal ulcers, and strictures, in 194,527 hospitalized veterans over a 14-year period, using computerized hospital records [12]. Although patients with esophageal ulcers or strictures were older than those with uncomplicated esophagitis, no particular temporal pattern could be established consistently.

In a large multicenter study including 1253 centers from Germany, Austria, and Switzerland, designed to look at the outcome for patients with GERD. Risk factor analysis was performed for 5289 patients with erosive reflux disease or NERD [28, 31]. Small number of erosive diseases are in the population with a higher level of education and the presence of *Helicobacter pylori*.

The association of a longer duration of symptoms with erosive esophagitis compared to some cases of NERD may complicate erosive disease.

Another study reported results for 51,311 patients over 15 years [32]. In most cases, Barrettt's esophagus peak arrived at the seventh to ninth decades. In 101 patients, there was no change in the length of BE. The authors showed that this happens more often in male patients aged 60, who had a follow-up endoscopy in a follow-up of 7.4 years.

NERD and erosive disease are part of the dilatation of intracellular spaces of esophageal epithelium confirmed on pH monitoring with results as follow: 38 patients with GERD and 22 with NERD. Early pathophysiological marker of esophageal damage is dilatation of intracellular spaces. Therapy with 40 mg omeprazole resulted in 97% complete recovery after 6 months in NERD and GERD [33]. High-grade dysplasia or esophageal adenocarcinoma can be prevented after using PPI therapy in patients with low -grade dysplasia. PPI therapy should be started after stratification by year within 2 years of definitive diagnosis (our results). LGD can be developed in case of delayed therapy with PPI.

This study confirms our observation that fewer patients with BE developed dysplasia after the introduction of PPI therapy in Australia in 1989. We postulated that the incidence of dysplasia was influenced by powerful acid suppression that reduced esophageal acid exposure.

El-Serag and Sonnenberg raported the relationship between the midle forms of erosive oesopahgitis, oesophageal ulcers and strictures, in 194527 hospitalized veterans over a 14-year period, using computerized hospital records [34]. In patients with Barret's oesophagus increased epithelial proliferation is step from dysplasia to adenocarcinoma.

Barrett's esophagus (BE) was found in 11% of our GERD patients [35]. No evidence of completely reverses the length of Barret's osophagus [36, 37].

It is very important to emphasize that anticecretory therapy and using cyclooxygenase 2 (COX-2) inhibitors can prevent development of adenocarcionoma [36]. Overexpression of COX-2 inhibits apoptosis, allowing cancer to grow, and COX-2 inhibitors can help ensure that cancer cells die [38]. At the gene level, COX-2 inhibitors can reduce inflammatory factors [39].

In another study was reported that from 350 patients, only 111 patients developed HGD or adenocarcinoma. It should be noted that study didn't have randomised controlled trial [29, 40]. Low-grade of dysplasia has atipical cells and active inflammation influenced in it [5, 35].

High-grade dysplasia was associated with macroscopic markers: severe esophagitis, nodularity, Barrett's ulcer or stricture [41].

In another study, the time of the start of PPI use in patients with BE was recorded. The degree of acid reduction was not measured. Also, the doses were not reduced, and this therapy was used for a long time, even though the symptoms of the disease were controlled [2]. Cancer risk for a given patient with BE is lower than previously estimated [23]. Risk factors for the progression of BE to EAC include the increasing degree of dysplasia, increasing age, increasing BE segment length, male sex, and smoking, among others [42].

The degree of dysplasia has been directly related to segment length. The greater the length of the BE segment, the more dysplasia we have [25].

However, when the BE develops, its length generally does not change, so the short-segment BE normally remains short even in the context of continuous exposure of the esophagus to acid. Actually, when we have BE with a short segment, its length does not change much even though it is under the influence of acid [18].

Dysplasia and adenocarcinoma are complications of long and short BE, and are treated similarly [27]. For that more, 20% have an improvement in intestinal metaplasia, but more than 50% had an improvement in patients with low-grade dysplasia. These findings are of great importance in the clinical management of patients with BE, especially given the widespread use of experimental ablative therapies aimed at achieving a similar goal. When we have treated gastroesophageal reflux, we have permission from the EU. Many errors have been minimized through biopsies according to the protocols, the sessions of two biopsies with an output of about 6 months, systematization of regression, so that the biopsy sample was the mucosa of the cardia. It is possible that IM will spontaneously regress to normal tissue without treatment. Additionally, these findings have importance in the clinical management of BE using ablative therapies.

Based on the literature, IM or dysplasia was known after PPI therapy. Intestinal metaplasia was lost in 39% of SSBE patients and 10% of LSBE. Female gender, absence of hiatal hernia, and shorter Barrett'length associated with loss of IM.

But Sampliner and others [43] suggested that follow up every 2 to 3 years in BE if no dysplasia after two endoscopies. If no change endoscopy should be done every year; in patients with LGD, they recommended every 6 months for the first year.

Author Sharma et al. reported in a multicenter study of LGD history; 35% had intermittent LGD; from the total of 1376 patients incidence of dysplasia was 4.3% every year; 7.3% was prevalence at presentation [44].

After medical therapy LGD had a regression. Our advice is that patients with intestinal dysplasia to follow up with proximal endoscopy every year. Patients with dysplasia should have every 3-month gastroscopic examination.

The goals for treating patients with BE are as follows:

1. Reduce gastroesophageal reflux

2. Regression or elimination of intestinal metaplasia

3. Reduce progression from dysplasia to cancer.

Shaheen et al. [45] Surgical antireflux procedures are highly effective at reducing gastroesophageal reflux episodes, healing esophagitis, and decreasing the symptoms associated with reflux. It is logical, therefore, to consider their application in the setting of BE to reduce the risk of progression to cancer.

To achieve the first goal of treatment for patients with BE the therapy had not guided by symptoms. Patients should have 24-hour PH monitoring. The author Castell et al. [46] reported an evening dose of H2 receptor antagonist in addition to the twice-daily dose of PPI. Better no therapy compared with incomplete therapy. Finally, gastric PH should be PH =7 with therapy.

Second and third goals therapy are to eliminate IM, to prevent dysplasia and cancer. Despite regular therapy, this did not cause IM regression [47, 48].

Langergren et al. reported the patients who have had symptoms like heartburn and regurgitation have been at risk for adenocarcinoma of the esophagus 8-fold more compared with patients without symptoms [49].

They concluded that treatment did not prevent dysplasia. Some studies had emphasized this issue. There was no reduction in the length of BE despite therapy with 60 mg lansoprazole once a day, almost 3 years [18].

Malesci et al. have shown reducing from length from 4.5 to 2.1 cm with therapy for acid suppression [50]. These studies have demonstrated the difficulties to replicate the impressive decreased length of BE. With PPI therapy twice daily arrived total control of esophageal acid but just in a series of 9 patients. The length of BE was from 7.2 to 5.2 cm (with $P < 0.0001$) [5]. The use of ranitidine 150 mg twice daily compared with omeprazole 40 mg showed a minimal decrease in segment length in BE. Histamine blockers are not effective in decreasing in the length of BE compared with omeprazole [12].

The conclusion are as follow:

1. The course of BE and mainly of GERD patients may be improved by therapy.

2. Improving appears to be higher in cases with SSBE and in absence of a hiatal hernia.

3. The effect of PPI in decreasing cases with LGD shows that this microscopic evidence was not irreversible.

4. We found that PPI therapy is very beneficial in preventing the development of low-grade dysplasia in BE.

Conflict of interest

The authors declare no conflict of interest.

Author details

Zaim Gashi[1,2], Arjeta Gashi[3] and Fadil Sherifi[2]*

1 UBT College, Prishtina, Republic of Kosova

2 UCCK, Clinic of Gastroenterology and Hepatology, Prishtina, Republic of Kosova

3 PharmItalia, Prishtina, Republic of Kosova

*Address all correspondence to: drfsh038@gmail.com

References

[1] Nebel OT, Fornes ME, Castell DO. Symptomatic gastresophageal reflux: Incidence and precipitating factors. American Journal of Digestive Diseases. 1976;**21**(11):953-956

[2] DeMeester TR, Johnson LF, Joseph GJ, Toscano MS, Hall AW, Skinner DB. Patterns of gastresophageal reflux in health and disease. Annals of Surgery. 1976;**184**(4):459-470

[3] Nandurkar S, Talley NJ. Epidemiology and natural history of reflux disease. Baillieres Best Practice and Research in Clinical Gastroenterology. 2000;**14**(5):743-757

[4] Hunt RH, Tytgat GH, Malfertheiner P, et al. Whistler summary: The slow rate of rapid progress. Journal of Clinical Gastroenterology. 2007;**41**(6):539-545

[5] Eros B et al. Helicobacter pylori reduce the risk of Barrett's esophagus: A meta analysis and systematic review. Helicobacter. 2018;**23**(4):el12504

[6] Vakil N. The frontiers of reflux disease. Digestive Diseases and Sciences. 2006;**51**(11):1887-1895

[7] Dean BB, Aguilar D, Johnson LF, et al. The relationship between the prevalence of nighttime gastresophageal reflux disease and disease severity. Digestive Diseases and Sciences. In press

[8] DeMeester TR, Bonavina L, Albertucci M. Nissen fundoplication for gastresophageal reflux disease: Evaluation of primary reflux in 100 consecutive patients. Annals of Surgery. 1986;**204**:9-20

[9] Spechler SJ. Epidemiology and natural history of gastresophageal reflux disease. Digestion. 1992;**51**(Supplement 1):24-29

[10] Smith JL, Opekun AR, Larkai E, Graham DY. Sensitivity of esophageal mucosa to pH in gastresophageal reflux disease. Gastroenterology. 1989;**96**(3):683-689

[11] Barrett's Esophagus. In Wikipedia. 4 Mar 2023. Available from: https://en.wikipedia.org/wiki/Barrett%27s_esophagus

[12] Jürgens S, Meyer F, Spechler SJ, Souza R. The role of bile acids in the neoplastic progression of Barrett's esophagus - a short representative overview; Review. Z Gastroenterol. Sep 2012;**50**(9):1028-1034. DOI: 10.1055/s-0032-1312922. Epub 2012 Sep 10. PMID: 22965634

[13] Campos GM, Peters JH, DeMeester TR, et al. The pattern of esophageal acid exposure in gastresophageal reflux disease influences the severity of the disease. Archives of Surgery. 1999;**134**(8):882-888

[14] Penagini R, Schoeman MN, Dent J, et al. Motor events underlying gastro-esophageal reflux in ambulant patients with reflux esophagitis. Neurogastroenterology and Motility. 1996;**8**(2):131-141

[15] Kulig M, Nocon M, Vieth M, et al. Risk factors of gastresophageal reflux disease: Methodology and first epidemiological results of the ProGERD study. Journal of Clinical Epidemiology. 2004;**57**:580-589

[16] Labenz J, Jaspersen D, Kulig M, et al. Risk factors for erosive esophagitis: A multivariate analysis based on the ProGERD study initiative. The American Journal of Gastroenterology. 2004;**99**:1652-1656

[17] Cameron AJ, Lomboy CT. Barrett's esophagus: Age, prevalence, and extent of columnar epithelium. Gastroenterology. 1992;**103**:1241-1245

[18] Calabrese C, Bortolotti M, Fabbri A, et al. Reversibility of GERD ultrastructural alterations and relief of symptoms after omeprazole treatment. The American Journal of Gastroenterology. 2005;**100**:537-542

[19] Calabrese C, Fabbri A, Bortolotti M, et al. Dilated intercellular spaces as a marker of esophageal damage: Comparative results in gastro-esophageal reflux disease with or without bile reflux. Alimentary Pharmacology & Therapeutics. 2003;**18**:525-532

[20] Ross-Innes CS et al. Evaluation of a minimally invasive cell sampling device coupled with assessment of trefoil factor 3 expression for diagnosing Barrett's esophagus: A multi-center case-control study. PLoS Medicine. **12**:e1001780

[21] Louie BE, Kapur S, Blitz M, Farivar AS, Vallières E, Aye RW. Length and pressure of the reconstructed lower esophageal sphincter is determined by both crural closure and Nissen fundoplication. Journal of Gastrointestinal Surgery. 2013;**17**:236-243

[22] Fennerty MB. Barrett's-related esophageal cancer: Has the final hurdle been cleared, now paving the way for human chemoprevention trials? Gastroenterology. 2002;**122**:1172-1175

[23] Falk GW. Barrett's esophagus. Gastroenterology. 2002;**122**:1569-1591

[24] Gashi Z. Dysplastic changes in esophageal reflux in hiatal hernia with esophageal burden and carcinoma. PHD thesis, Skopje-Macedonia. 2013

[25] Peters FTM, Ganesh S, Kuipers EJ, et al. Effect of elimination of acid reflux on epithelial cell proliferative activity of Barrett esophagus. Scandinavian Journal of Gastroenterology. 2000;**12**:1239-1244

[26] Isolauri J, Luostarinen M, Isolauri E, Reinikainen P, Viljakka M, Keyrilainen O. Year follow-up of 60 patients natural course of gastresophageal reflux disease: 17-22. The American Journal of Gastroenterology. 1997;**92**:37-41

[27] Ouatu-Lascar R, Fitzgerald RC, Triadafilopoulos G. Differentiation and proliferation in Barrett's esophagus and the effects of acid suppression. Gastroenterology. 1999;**117**:327-335

[28] McDougall NI, Johnston BT, Collins JS, McFarland RJ, Love AH. Years after diagnosis disease progression in gastro-esophageal reflux disease as determined by repeat esophageal pH monitoring and endoscopy 3 to 4.5. European Journal of Gastroenterology & Hepatology. 1997;**9**:1161-1167

[29] Fennerty MB, Triadafilopoulos G. Barrett's related adenocarcinoma: Is chemoprevention a potential option? The American Journal of Gastroenterology. 2001;**96**:2302-2305

[30] Bajbouj M, Reichenberger J, Neu B, et al. A prospective multicenter clinical and endoscopic follow-up study of patients with gastresophageal reflux disease. Zeitschrift für Gastroenterologie. 2005;**43**:1303-1307

[31] Klinkenberg-Knol EC, Nelis F, Dent J, et al. Long-term omeprazole treatment in resistant gastresophageal reflux disease: Efficacy, safety, and influence on gastric mucosa. Gastroenterology. 2000;**118**:661-669

[32] Garrido SA, Guerrero Igea FJ, Lepe Jimenez JA, Perianes HC. Clinical features and endoscopic progression of gastresophageal reflux disease. Revista

Española de Enfermedades Digestivas. 2003;**95**:712-716

[33] Brossard E, Monnier P, Ollyo J-B. Serious complications - stenosis, ulcers and Barrett's epithelium – Develop in 21.6% of patients with erosive reflux esophagitis. Gastroenterology. 1991;**100**:A36

[34] El-Serag HB, Sonnenberg A. Associations between different forms of gastro-esophageal reflux disease. Gut. 1997;**41**(5):594-599

[35] Schmidt HG, Riddell RH, Walther B, et al. Dysplasia in Barrett's esophagus. Journal of Cancer Research and Clinical Oncology. 1985;**110**:145-152

[36] Xu X. Cyclooxygenase-2 inhibitors in cancer treatment and prevention, a recent development. Anticancer Drugs. 2002;**13**:127-137. DOI: 10.1097/00001813-200202000-00003

[37] Sampliner RE, Fennerty B, Garewal HS. Reversal of Barrett's esophagus with acid suppression and multipolar electrocoagulation: Preliminary results. Gastrointestinal Endoscopy. Nov 1996;**44**(5):532-535

[38] Lindsey. Heather:COX-2 Inhibitors for Cancer Prevention & Treatment. Oncology Times. Apr 2002;**24**(4):52-54. DOI: 10.1097/01.COT.0000285556.13978.51

[39] Li A, Jiang M, et al. Combined chemotherapy with cyclooxygenase-2 (COX-2) inhibitors in treating human cancers: Recent advancement. Biomedicine & Pharmacotherapy. Sep 2020;**129**:110389

[40] Chen L, Hu C, Gaboury L, et al. Proliferative activity in Barrett's esophagus before and after antireflux surgery. Annals of Surgery. 2001;**234**:172-180

[41] Lybus C et al. Barrett's esophagus: Macroscopic markers and the prediction of dysplasia and adenocarcinoma. Journal of Gastroenterology and Hepatology. May 2003;**18**(5):526-533. DOI: 10.1046/j.1440-1746.2003.02965.x

[42] Gopal DV, Lieberman DA, Magaret N, Fennerty MB, Sampliner RE, Garewal HS, et al. Risk factors for dysplasia in patients with Barrett's esophagus (BE): Results from a multicenter consortium. Digestive Diseases and Sciences. 2003;**48**:1537-1541

[43] Sampliner RE, The Practice Parameters Committee of the American College of Gastroenterology. Practice guidelines on the diagnosis, surveillance, and therapy of Barrett's esophagus. The American Journal of Gastroenterology. 1998;**93**:1028-1032

[44] Sharma P, Falk GW, Weston AP, Reker D, Johnston M, Sampliner RE. Dysplasia and cancer in a large multicenter cohort of patients with Barrett's esophagus. Clinical Gastroenterology and Hepatology. 2006;**4**:566-572

[45] Shaheen Nicholas J, Falk Gary W, Iyer Prasad G, Souza Rhonda F, Yadlapati Rena H, Sauer Bryan G, et al. Clinical Guidelines, Diagnosis and Management of Barrett's Esophagus: An Updated ACG Guideline. The American Journal of Gastroenterology. 2022;**117**(4):559-587. DOI: 10.14309/ajg.0000000000001680

[46] D.O. Castell: What Is the Short-Term Reproducibility of the Results of 24-h pH Measurement in GER?, OESO Books, Philadephia, 1994

[47] Ortiz A, Martinez de Haro LF, Parrilla P, et al. Conservative treatment versus antireflux Surg in Barrett's oesophagus: Long-term results of a prospective study. The British Journal of Surgery. 1996;**83**:274-278

[48] Sampliner RE, Garewal HS, Fennerty MB, Aickin M. Lack of impact of therapy on extent of Barrett's esophagus in 67 patients. Digestive Diseases and Sciences. 1990;**35**:93-96

[49] Lagergren J, Bergstrom R, Lindgren A, Nyren O. Symptomatic gastresophageal reflux as a risk factor for esophageal adenocarcinoma. The New England Journal of Medicine. 1999;**340**:825-831

[50] Malesci A, Savarino V, Zentilin P, et al. Partial regression of Barrett's esophagus by long-term therapy with high-dose omeprazole. Gastrointestinal Endoscopy. 1996;**44**:700-705